P a r t i a l   V i e w

Partial View

An Alzheimer's Journal

TEXT BY CARY SMITH HENDERSON
PHOTOGRAPHS BY NANCY ANDREWS

Edited by Jackie Henderson Main, Ruth D. Henderson, and Nancy Andrews

Foreword by Lonnie D. Kliever
Introduction by Ruth D. Henderson
Afterword by Sarah Vann Wyne

SOUTHERN METHODIST UNIVERSITY PRESS

Dallas

Copyright © 1998 by Cary Smith Henderson and Nancy Andrews
All rights reserved
First edition, 1998

Requests for permission to reproduce material from this work should be sent to:

Permissions
Southern Methodist University Press
PO Box 750415
Dallas, TX 75275-0415

LIBRARY OF CONGRESS CATALOGING-IN-PUBLICATION DATA

Henderson, Cary Smith.
    Partial view : an Alzheimer's journal / text by Cary Smith Henderson ; photographs by Nancy Andrews ; edited by Jackie Henderson Main, Ruth D. Henderson, and Nancy Andrews ; foreword by Lonnie D. Kliever ; introduction by Ruth D. Henderson ; afterword by Sarah Vann Wyne.
       p.   cm.
    ISBN 0-87074-438-0 (pbk.)
    1. Henderson, Cary Smith—Health. 2. Alzheimer's disease—Patients—United States—Biography. I. Main, Jackie Henderson. II. Henderson, Ruth D. III. Andrews, Nancy, 1963– . IV. Title.
RC523.2.H46   1998
362.1' 96831' 0092—dc21   98-38368
[B]

Design by Tom Dawson Graphic Design, Dallas, Texas
Printed by Blanks Color Imaging, Inc., Dallas, Texas

Printed in the United States of America on acid-free paper
10 9 8 7 6 5 4 3 2 1

All of the photographs in this book were made from March 1994 through August 1995. Many family members, friends and medical professionals appear in these photographs on the following pages:

12 wife Ruth Henderson
14 Ruth Henderson
16 grandson Elijah Main
24 Elijah Main
26 daughter-in-law Joann Henderson, grandchildren Max Henderson, Anna Henderson, Elijah Main, daughter Jackie Main, son-in-law David Main, Ruth Henderson, son Jim Henderson
28 Ruth Henderson
34 Jackie Main, Elijah Main, Ruth Henderson
38 Ruth Henderson, Elijah Main
44 Elijah Main, Ruth Henderson, Jackie Main, Jim Henderson, Anna Henderson, Max Henderson
54 Cary with George Beckerman and Thomas Reeve at the Duke Medical Center support group for people with Alzheimer's disease
60 at Duke, Ruth Henderson, Sarah Vann Wyne, Dr. Nancy Earl
62 Dr. Nancy Earl
68 Ruth Henderson, Joann Henderson, Anna Henderson, Jim Henderson
75 Elijah Main
80 Ruth Henderson
84 Ruth Henderson

This book is dedicated to
Cary Smith Henderson and Jackie Henderson Main,
father and daughter. Together they dreamed the reality of this book.
Cary, alone, shared his world of Alzheimer's and then Jackie, with Cary
no longer available, helped to turn their dream into a reality.

RUTH D. HENDERSON

The best thing to do about this is just not worry about it.
Be happy with the partial view or whatever else is partial, everything is partial.

CARY SMITH HENDERSON

Contents

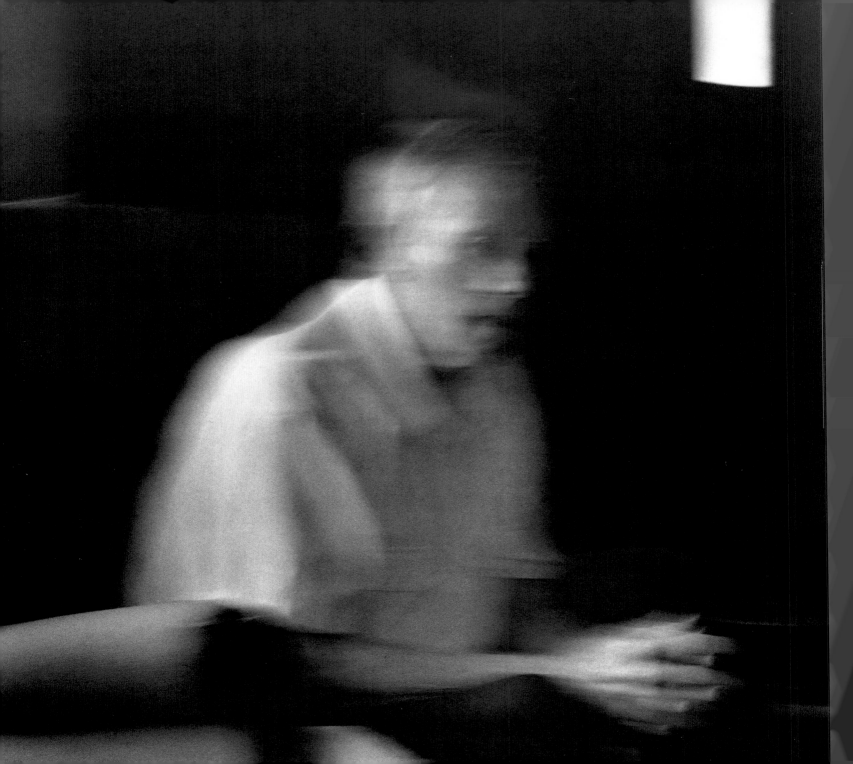

NARRATIVES OF ILLNESS have become a staple of talk shows, best-seller lists, and medical school classrooms. These stories told by celebrities or unknowns who have struggled or are struggling with some form of disease or disability have broken down the walls of silence and shame that often surround their condition. They have provided a map and a destination for those who must travel into the world of the sick—patients and professionals, families and friends—offering information and inspiration for their journeys. At their best, these "wounded storytellers" have shown others how to live and even how to die.

Most of the illness groups are well represented in this remarkable literature. Life stories dealing with cancer, cardiovascular disease, and AIDS, as well as chronic fatigue syndrome, depression, and schizophrenia, would fill a small library. One disease remains virtually unreported among such narratives of illness—Alzheimer's disease. This lack is not for want of travelers into this shadow world of illness. About four million Americans, including half of the million six hundred thousand Americans in nursing homes, suffer from Alzheimer's. Very few of them have even tried to tell their stories.

The reasons for their silence are heartbreakingly obvious: there are no survivors or happy endings for persons with this disease. Barring a medical breakthrough, there is no cure for this remorseless disease. The best that a new line of antidementia drugs can promise is slowing down the irreversible decline of Alzheimer's patients. But there is a more telling reason why there are so few map-makers in the Alzheimer's community. Alzheimer's patients are not able to remember enough about their former lives, about their current debility, even about how to put language together into sentences, to tell their stories. Given the difficulties of diagnosis and the resistance to disclosure, most patients slip into the world of the "deeply forgetful" without articulating what is happening to them.

xii

Cary Henderson was an exception. A brain shunt operation produced an early diagnosis which allowed him to do a number of things denied most Alzheimer's patients. He and his wife were able to take the trips they were saving for their retirement years. He was able to plan for the future and to participate in many of his own treatment decisions. Perhaps most important of all, Henderson was able to accumulate the "field notes" which here provide this unique insider's view of the world of Alzheimer's. He did not work alone in charting his course. He was joined by Nancy Andrews, whose photographic record of his journey lends vividness to

his story. Her images empower the words as surely as his words interpret the images.

Like many writers of illness narratives, Cary Henderson found that the act of recording his experiences was simultaneously a means of maintaining his own sense of self and of trying to help others in their struggle with Alzheimer's disease. Authors such as Elaine Scarry *(The Body in Pain)* and Arthur W. Frank *(The Wounded Storyteller)* have shown that seriously ill people are wounded not just in body but in voice. They need to become storytellers to recover the voices that illness and treatment often silence. Their narratives are a way of transcending bodily suffering and mental anguish and their stories are a way of reaching out and helping others. Their illness becomes the source of the potency of their stories, creating empathic bonds between themselves and their auditors. Wounded storytellers become wounded healers.

Nowhere is this need to tell and share stories more urgent and more difficult than in the world of Alzheimer's, where loss of voice is more than a metaphor of the powerlessness and isolation brought on by serious illness. Alzheimer's unravels a lifetime of cognitive development, steadily moving backward along the developmental path until only the most basic emotions and instincts are left. Memory goes first, then comprehension, finally language itself. Henderson's reach for language to document his experience was a way of humanizing that dehumanizing journey—rendering it more understandable to himself and therefore more bearable for those who must suffer its devastation directly or indirectly.

Henderson used the tools of a lifetime of training as a professional historian to tell his story—the narrative voice of firsthand testimony. Careless readers may miss the powerful message that comes through in his descriptions of panic, paranoia, anger, shame, wonder, gratitude, and sadness, most of which are rather ordinary and few of which are truly profound. But that failure will be the reader's and not the teller's fault. There *is* a powerful message in these sometimes rambling and repetitive notes from the underground. No poet or philosopher could describe the Alzheimer's world with greater force than Henderson's own words: "I just had a brilliant idea, but before I could push down the little recording mechanism, it was absolutely totally gone [7]. It's kinda nice to talk to a dog that you know is not going to talk back. And you can't make a mistake that way [13]. I'd like a larger world than I have right now [24]. Some time back, we used to be, I hesitate to say

the word, 'human beings' [35]. I'm not really sure Alzheimer's is a killer, in the usual sense of the word, it's a maimer. I'm sure, a maimer of—what did I say?— certainly a killer of people's thoughts [59]. I certainly have no right to criticize anybody, but I just hope that my family and friends do realize that being an Alzheimer's person is—just a little bit of hell [83]."

In other words, there is a remarkable connection between the *form* and *content* of Henderson's ruminations which tells us much about the Alzheimer's world. For one thing, there is no time line in Henderson's reflections. They happen in a timeless or a time-fractured world where time as easily flows backward as forward, as easily creeps like a snail or sweeps like the wind. But this absence reflects more than a loss of clock or calendar time. Henderson's words and images convey no vital memory or hope for the future. There is occasional recognition and surprise which betrays a semblance of enduring memory and hope, but nothing that commemorates a memorable past or anticipates a worthwhile future. "No two days and no two moments are the same. You can't build on experience. You can maybe guess what's going to happen a little while from now —minutes from now, hours from now—we don't know what to expect [47]."

xiii

This absence of a narrative time line reflects the progressive loss of the ability to choose, sort, and arrange all the information that the human environment presents. Henderson marks the loss of these organizing powers in the most elemental of human activities. Conversation becomes a treacherous minefield of missed connections and muddled words. "I can't think of things to say before somebody's already said it and they've superseded what I had to say. The words get tangled very easily and I get frustrated when I can't think of a word. Every time I converse with somebody, there's always some word I can't remember [18]." Reading is reduced to a blur of half-recognized marks on the page. "Reading's almost impossible. For one thing—things don't stand still. Words don't stand still. It appears to me that it's wavering. I can't pin it down—the words—they can be over yonder and over yonder and I can't catch them [23]." Even opening a can of dog food becomes a test of concentration and finding the way back home a trial-and-error ordeal. "There's a lot of things that happen when I'm walking the dog. This morning—it was rather embarrassing—to be living in Harrisonburg, Virginia, now for a long long time—many many years—we've been living in the same place for a long long time, and I still have trouble knowing where things are [48]."

Despite these losses, there are reminders of the deeper reserves of the human spirit. Henderson remains responsive to experiences of beauty. He finds comfort and pleasure in music. "I can just listen to music and feel that I'm doing something that I just love to do. I can't make music anymore, but I can certainly use it for my own intentions—which are just to be beautiful [42]." He enjoys the changes of the seasons and the marvels of nature. "I still pick up leaves, probably the same ones I had before. I love the fall colors. I pick 'em up anyhow, whether I have them or not. Every year it seems like they're prettier and prettier. I appreciate them a lot more now than I did a few years ago [77]." Henderson also remains sensitive to the needs of others. He worries about the toll on his caregivers and reaches out to his Alzheimer's companions. "I think that is the one thing that is the most difficult about Alzheimer's— is loving, continuously and without qualms, without holding anything back—it's a matter of trust. I think probably, though, that anybody who is a caregiver to an Alzheimer's patient, their patience is just going to be continually bothered [65]."

Finally, a cumulative sense of the mystery of the self shines through Henderson's "anecdotal career of an Alzheimer's patient." That self is directly visible in occasional moments of startling lucidity and profundity, but indirectly present like some phantom limb in every recital. Some *person* has these experiences of confusion and alienation—someone *knows* that he forgets, *recognizes* his stupidity, *regrets* his anger, *realizes* that he is lost. The core of selfhood—self-awareness—remains, at least in the middle course of the disease.

Like those intrepid explorers of old who traveled to the edge of the world, Cary Henderson had the courage to observe and communicate the increasing wreckage of his world and his identity. He has left behind a bare-bones, soul-searching record that plumbs the terror and beauty of this human condition. With the help of the revealing and haunting photography of Nancy Andrews, he simply takes us *into* the world of Alzheimer's with an immediacy that is more informative than a medical textbook, more challenging than an ethics case study, and more inspiring than a religious memoir. He thereby snatches some comfort and even some dignity for himself and for all those faded selves who cannot speak for themselves.

LONNIE D. KLIEVER
Professor of Religious Studies
Southern Methodist University
Dallas, Texas
August 1998

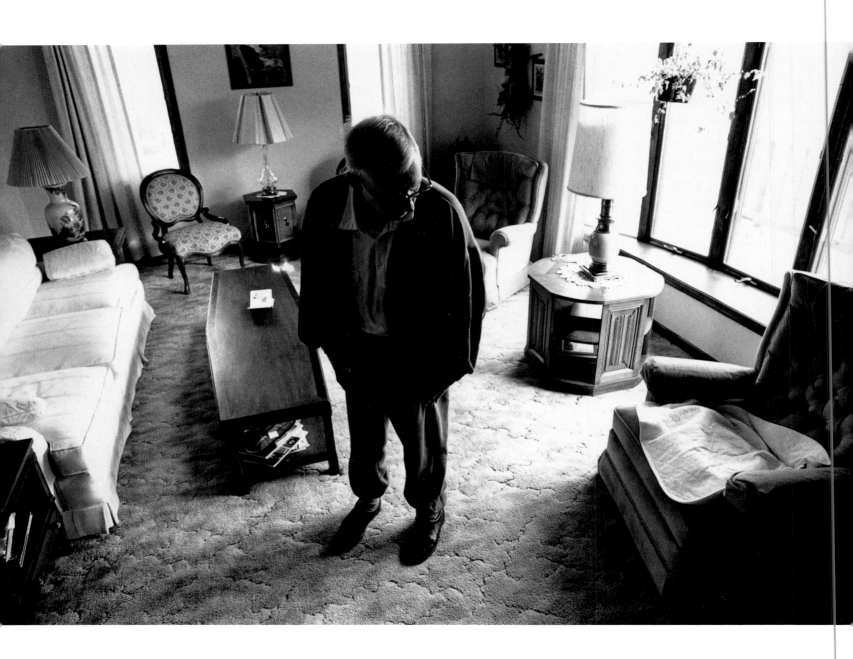

WRITING AN INTRODUCTION to a book should be the privilege of the author, but the steady and relentless encroachment of Alzheimer's disease has silenced Cary's voice forever. Now sixty-eight years old, he still lives, but only in the sense of a beating heart and lungs that continue to take in air. The man who spoke of his efforts to live with Alzheimer's disease and who wanted to help others understand more about the disease now lies mute and helpless in a nursing home bed, unable to do the smallest thing for himself. Yet some tiny spark still lives within him—when I told him that his book would be published, Cary's eyes filled with tears, tears that I choose to believe were tears of joy. This project meant everything to him at the time he dictated his musings and when he sat and listened to Nancy Andrews, our good friend and photographer; Jackie Main, our daughter; and me, as we worked to edit his thoughts into a readable book.

Cary Henderson was a Georgia boy whose family moved south to Jacksonville, Florida, just before the beginning of World War II. He was the first of his family to achieve higher education and he became a college professor with a Ph.D. in history from Duke University. We married very young and made this journey into academia together. We had three children,

Introduction

Jim, Tim, and Jackie, while Cary taught at the secondary and junior college level and worked on his doctorate. During these early years Cary also continued to develop the many interests which added so much richness and meaning to his life. He loved music and had a good baritone voice which he used to sing in church choirs and musicals on the college and community level. Although he was a rather shy and diffident man, he came to life on a stage with local theater groups. He also played the cornet, from high school through to the community band of Harrisonburg, Virginia. Another passion was photography, which he perfected to a semiprofessional level, photographing weddings, college sports events, dog shows, and nature, and making portraits of students. Cary also had a strong belief in volunteerism. He would drive the sick to medical appointments, ring the bell at Christmastime for the Salvation Army, work with the local area food bank, and as a lifetime member of Kiwanis he was secretary of his local club for eight years.

This gratifying life began to slow down in the early 1980s, with Cary giving up on one activity and then another as he searched for answers to disabling headaches and vision problems. In 1985, at the age of fifty-five, Cary had a CAT scan which led to a diagnosis of prob-

able normal pressure hydrocephalus because the scan showed abnormally large ventricular spaces, and we were told that he could have a shunt operation which would alleviate the fluid build-up in the ventricles of the brain and correct the condition. I asked the neurosurgeon who was to perform the operation if Alzheimer's disease was a possibility, and he took the precaution of taking a small segment of brain tissue during the operation for a biopsy. The tissue showed the characteristic plaques and tangles of Alzheimer's disease and I was told that Cary had a terminal illness; he could live for two more years or twenty more years, but there was no treatment and his condition would steadily worsen. I made the decision to delay telling Cary until he had recovered from the shunt operation, which had been unnecessary, as it turned out. About two months later, on a Sunday morning just before we were to leave for church, Cary said he wanted to go back to the hospital at the University of Virginia and tell them that his headaches were no better. I knew the time had come to tell him the truth, and even now, thirteen years later, I feel it was the most difficult thing I've ever done. I had decided that it was kinder to be definite and I told him there was no mistake, the biopsy had provided a certain diagnosis usually not available until an autopsy is done at the time of death. We never got to church that morning; we stayed in the kitchen for hours, crying and hugging each other and making plans. As Cary struggled to accept his fate, I realized again what a special person I was married to. We decided right then and there that as soon as possible we would do all the traveling we had planned for our retirement, do it while Cary was still able to enjoy it. This decision led to trips to Europe, the Pacific Northwest, and New England and Nova Scotia.

In the two years between Cary's diagnosis and his retirement, he continued to teach part-time, thanks to the understanding and compassion of his department head. But by the end of the first semester of the second year, we all knew that it was over. Students were complaining about his inability to lecture; I had to grade his exams when he brought them home and looked at me helplessly; then, when I asked him how to figure the students' grades for the course, he couldn't tell me. He was asked to retire by May 1987 and he was given a sabbatical semester to finish off his teaching career. During that semester, Cary occupied himself doing research for a book he believed would be an original contribution to the field of American history, but nothing came of it despite his best efforts. This was

a very frustrating time for Cary; he was still able to read and write, although on a much reduced level, and while he knew he had Alzheimer's disease, he found it hard to understand and accept that he wasn't able to put his research together coherently.

The week after Cary cleaned out his office at James Madison University and brought all of his books and files back home, we experienced a disaster in the form of a house fire. Cary and I escaped from the house unharmed in the middle of the night, but we lost our two Yorkshire terriers and most of our possessions. The fire began in our kitchen trash can where Cary had discarded a cigar stub not thoroughly extinguished. A mistake to lay at the door of Alzheimer's disease or a mistake that could happen to anybody? The shock of the fire and our subsequent gypsy life in motels until the house was rebuilt caused a discernible increase in Cary's symptoms. He never drove a car again after the fire, he never wanted to smoke another cigar, and his ability to read and write decreased measurably.

During the first three years after Cary's diagnosis, we sought help from our local medical establishment— general practitioners, a neurologist, and a psychiatrist. Then, in 1988, we began to read of a new drug called THA or tacrine which was being tested as a treatment for Alzheimer's disease. I pursued this lead thanks to a great deal of urging from our son Jim. After rejections from two research centers, we connected with the Duke Memory Disorders Clinic and Cary became an experimental subject there early in 1989. He was especially valuable to the drug study since he was one of the few people in the country who was definitely diagnosed with Alzheimer's disease as a result of the biopsy done during his shunt operation. Our association with the wonderful, caring people there was a lifeline, a little spot of sunshine in the very bleak landscape of our lives. Cary's years at Duke were exciting in several ways. Being involved in the study gave him a feeling of importance and added some meaning to his life. The people at the Clinic treated us like close friends, and that is how we felt about them. We both enjoyed the frequent four-hundred-mile round trips and looked on them as mini-vacations. Cary responded well to the drug tacrine, which is now commercially known and marketed as Cognex. He felt better, more alert and more able to take care of himself. Cary was told at the Clinic that this drug was not a cure and that the disease would progress, but he could not help but feel hopeful.

It was during this period that Cary and Jackie began to talk about collaborating on a book about Alzheimer's disease. They talked about it on walks with Cary's dog Uni, his constant companion since she came into our lives right after the fire. They thought perhaps Jackie could interview Cary and write down his responses, but Cary found it hard to admit he couldn't do it himself.

We watched sorrowfully as Cary's ability to read and to write deteriorated. Reading and writing had been his vocation and avocation, and he was very despondent over these losses, even though tacrine was helping in general. He would sit for hours trying to read one page in a history book or he would practice writing at the kitchen table—struggling to make his scribbling legible. When we visited our friends Chris and Anthony LaForgia in New Jersey in the summer of 1991, Anthony told Cary that he used a pocket tape recorder to keep reminders and shopping lists, instead of writing things down, and he suggested that Cary try to use one. When we got back home to Virginia, the first thing Cary did was ask me to dial Jackie's number and he told her he had an answer to their book project—he would put his thoughts about Alzheimer's disease on a tape recorder. At first, he couldn't seem to generate any thoughts and Jackie had to ask him questions, sort of priming the pump, but very soon he just took off and "mused" or "philosophized" by himself. He wanted to be alone when he did his taping, so it was necessary to label the recorder and try to teach him to use it. Sometimes his dictation got lost—the tapes are full of instances where we can hear that he had just turned the recorder on after having said all kinds of marvelous, insightful things for several minutes before realizing that the machine wasn't turned on. When I began to transcribe his dictation, I was overwhelmed by his insight into his disease. I heard things that he had never said to me or to anyone. Cary has always been a reticent person; he has rarely been able to share his feelings and thoughts with others. Somehow, the tape recorder liberated his thinking—he didn't have to keep a "stiff upper lip" when he was by himself with just his recorder for a companion. We realized that he was giving us a picture of the world that is Alzheimer's disease.

Soon Cary announced proudly to the people at Duke that he was writing a book for people with Alzheimer's disease, to help them cope with the illness through the insight he had achieved by living with the disease. Cary kept the journal from the fall of 1991 to the summer of 1992 when he felt he had said all he was capable of. When he was finished he had used about forty tapes which were transcribed onto about three

hundred pages. I was asked to excerpt about six pages of Cary's journal for inclusion in a quarterly periodical called the *Duke Caregiver*. After this newsletter was published, we began to get calls from around the country from people who were intrigued and interested in what Cary had to say.

By this time Jackie, her husband David, their son Eli, Cary and I were living in a large converted two-family house in the country right outside of Harrisonburg. We all made the move in order to be able to take care of Cary ourselves and not have to place him in a nursing home.

When *The Washington Post* asked to do an article about Cary for their Health section, we were told they would send a staff photographer to our home. Cary loved Nancy Andrews immediately. Their mutual love of photography created a bond between them as Nancy worked with him to get her pictures. And something in Cary reached out to her. She cried when she realized that he could no longer handle a camera or even put on his own gloves. So, the stranger who came to photograph him left the next day as a family friend and potential partner in the creation of a book.

The book progressed during the next year, and Cary sat in on all the meetings as Jackie, Nancy and I worked on editing the huge amount of work he had done. During this same time, the story in *The Washington Post* led to another feature in *Better Homes and Gardens* and then to a CNN special on the disease, "The Long Good-bye." The program was filmed in the summer of 1995 and Cary was still able to react to some questions and walk with help.

Except for the CNN filming, 1995 was a bad year for Cary. He was hospitalized four times for various physical ailments, and each time his body and mind descended to a new plateau of functioning which finally led us to place him in a nursing home.

Cary hoped very strongly that his musings would be of use to others; that he could help those afflicted to live more fully and more at peace with their disease; and that he could help others understand what it feels like to have Alzheimer's disease. My family and I hope that his legacy will reach out to you.

RUTH D. HENDERSON
Harrisonburg, Virginia
August 1998

Partial View

I guess probably the best thing that ever happened to me was while I was with Alzheimer's is that my speech has not been impeded—it's still pretty good. I may not know all the time what I'm talking about, but I, damn it, still I can talk.

It's a sincere effort to get this off my chest. I never was quiet. When I hurt, I yell, which is what I've been doing for several years now, and it's food for thought, at least, an Alzheimer's picnic.

I'm taking it as one of my duties in trying to write this book, to sort of get people with Alzheimer's knowledgeable about what they can expect and what they can do, and of course, what they can't do.

Perhaps I can help somebody else understand the world that they are now forced to live in.

I would like to be somebody who could help understanding from the patient's point of view—what it is like to be an Alzheimer's patient.

It's somebody's version of hell and I guess I'll someday have to write a book about that, which is exactly what I am trying to do. To whoever can read it to you, if you need to be read to, I would be glad to sell you a copy of my little Bible of Alzheimer's—the anecdotal career of an Alzheimer's patient.

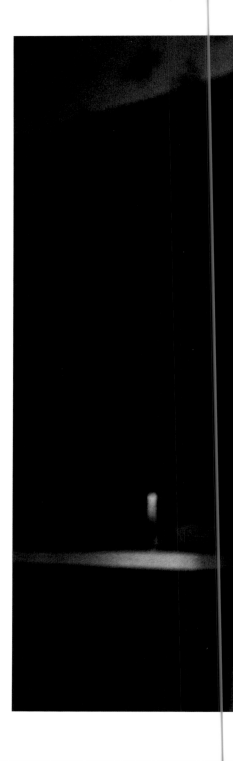

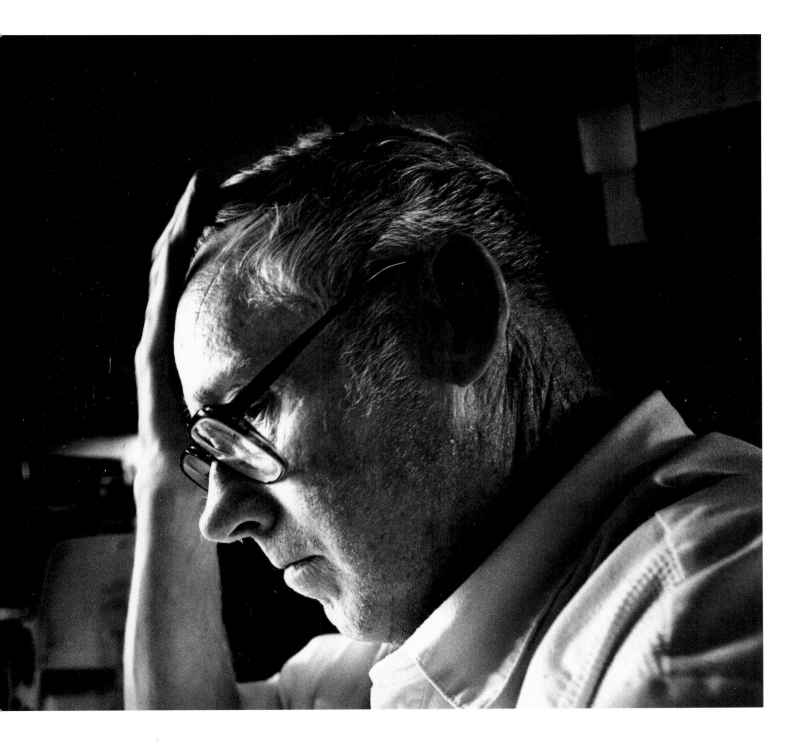

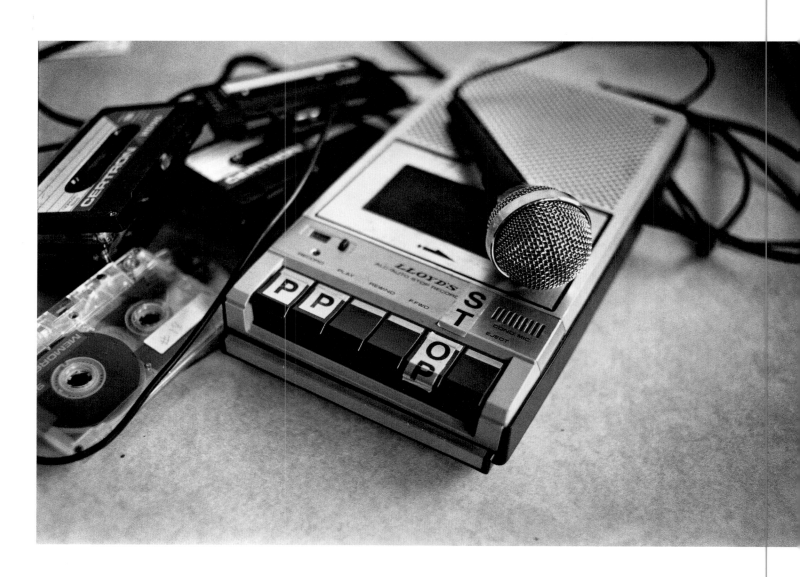

I would love to see some people with Alzheimer's not trying to stay in the shadows all the time but to say, damn it, we're people too. And we want to be talked to and respected as if we were honest to God real people.

So if you can get the ideas down, you can communicate better, you can keep your ideas long enough so somebody else can hear them, which may be a very valuable thing.

It's very much worth having—a memory device— an electronic memory device.

I still haven't mastered this, apparently very simple thing of—uh—pushing down the two sides to get the machine to work. Pushing two buttons ought to be the easiest thing on earth. I don't know, I must have another problem besides Alzheimer's. I don't know.

After a couple more mishaps I finally got the machine working. I suspect that for several minutes it hasn't been doing right, and of course, being me, I don't know what the heck I did wrong.

I just had a brilliant idea, but before I could push down the little recording mechanism, it was absolutely totally gone.

I do very seriously miss the things that I used to have.

I used to be able to talk to people and to walk without wondering if the pavement is actually there.

So many times I can't visualize things and I can't think through things, and it does get frustrating, and I'm not the type to take these things easily. I get mad. When I trip over something, I get mad. I do believe that Alzheimer's does include what your feet do and what your hands do, as well as what your brain does.

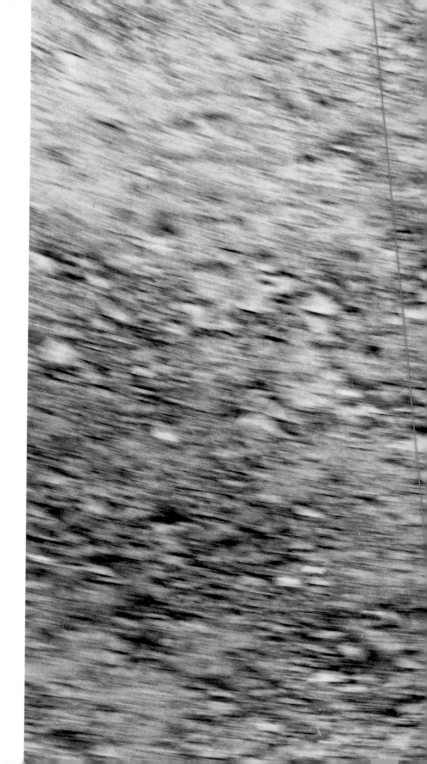

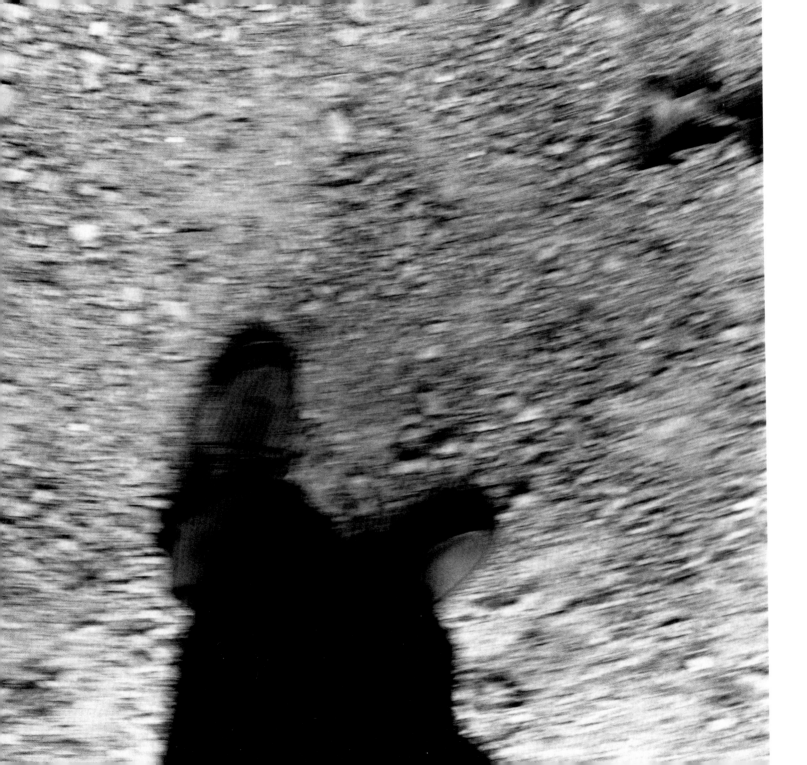

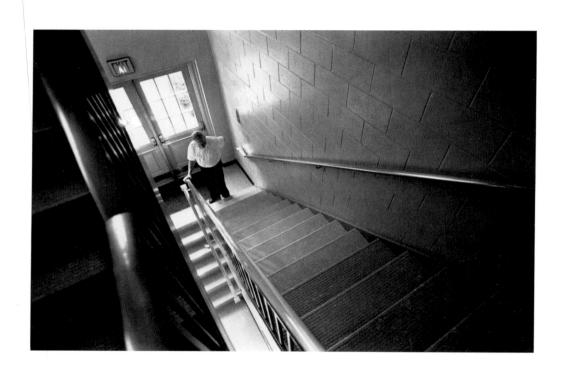

I'm scared to death of climbing stairs. Mainly because my feet don't go exactly where I think they want to go. To put it another way, I'm not really sure which way I want them to go. Alzheimer's kills a lot of instincts you once had.

I'm very tentative when I go up a stair, down a stair. I've got to hold on pretty tightly, then I'll go screaming meemies, the uncertainty of one's footage.

I'm very close to falling off—I'm doing something that's dangerous.

I get nervous on anything that's higher than a few inches.

It does get kind of serious. It's also maybe silly, because even if you're not about to fall down or something, you think you are. You feel that you are.

That's one of my bugaboos—I'm scared to death of going down stairs. And it's not a whole lot better going up stairs. You can't live on the bottom all the time, though.

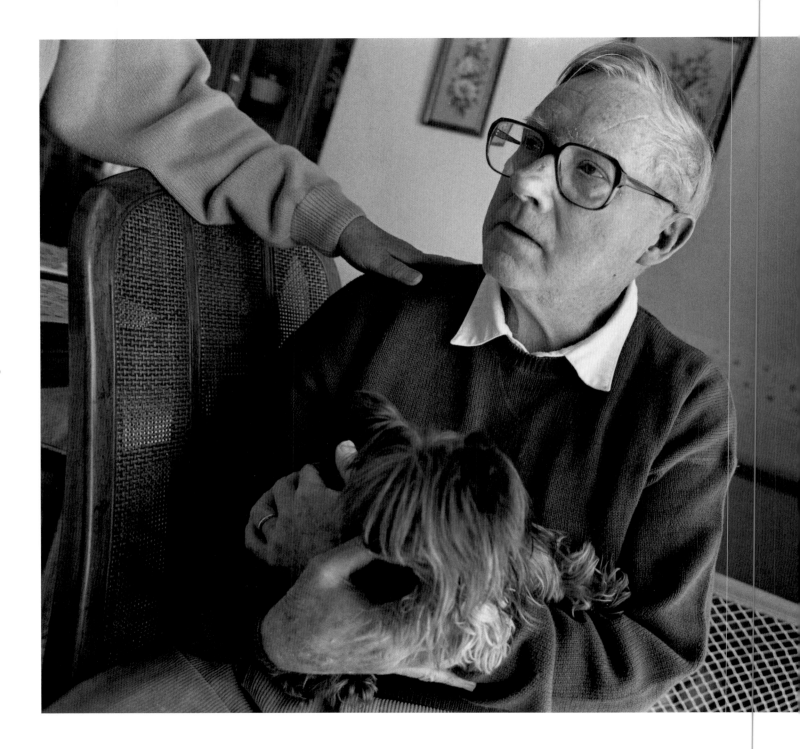

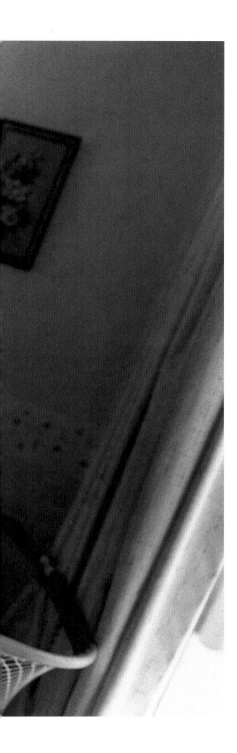

I sort of think that anybody with Alzheimer's could benefit by a friendly little dog. Somebody they can play with and talk to—it's kinda nice to talk to a dog that you know is not going to talk back. And you can't make a mistake that way.

But my dog is a small dog and it's not much for a seeing eye dog, or not very much to remember the things that I should. But she's very friendly. She doesn't talk, she doesn't remember things, but I love her anyhow. She gives me a lot of fun just watching her.

She's just a companion who's always there.

There are things I wish I could do, but on the other side, there are still things that I can do and I plan to hold on to them as long as I possibly can. Laughing is absolutely wonderful. A sense of humor is probably the most important valuable thing you can have when you have Alzheimer's.

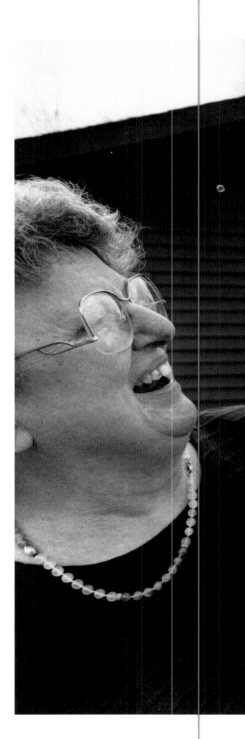

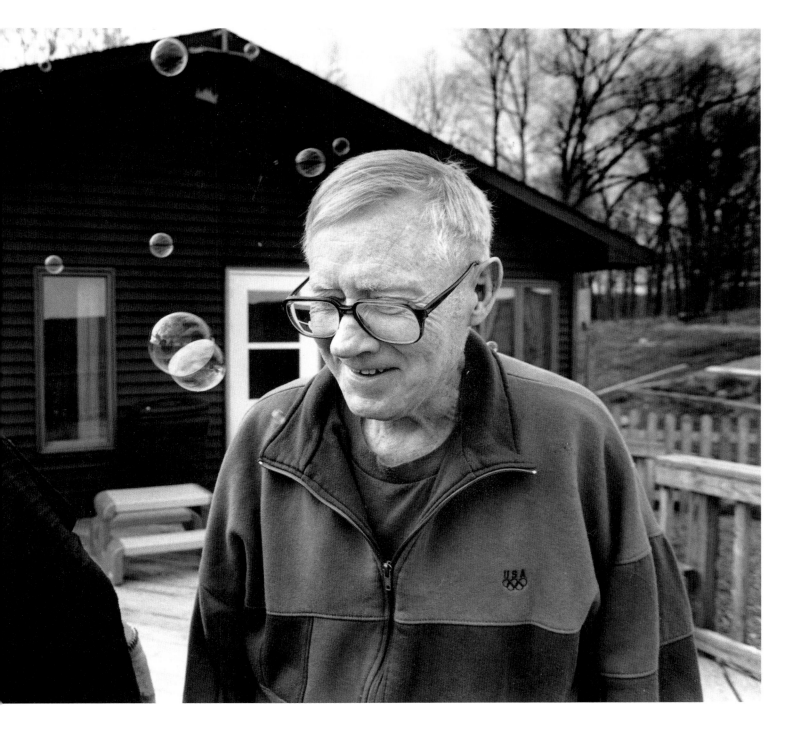

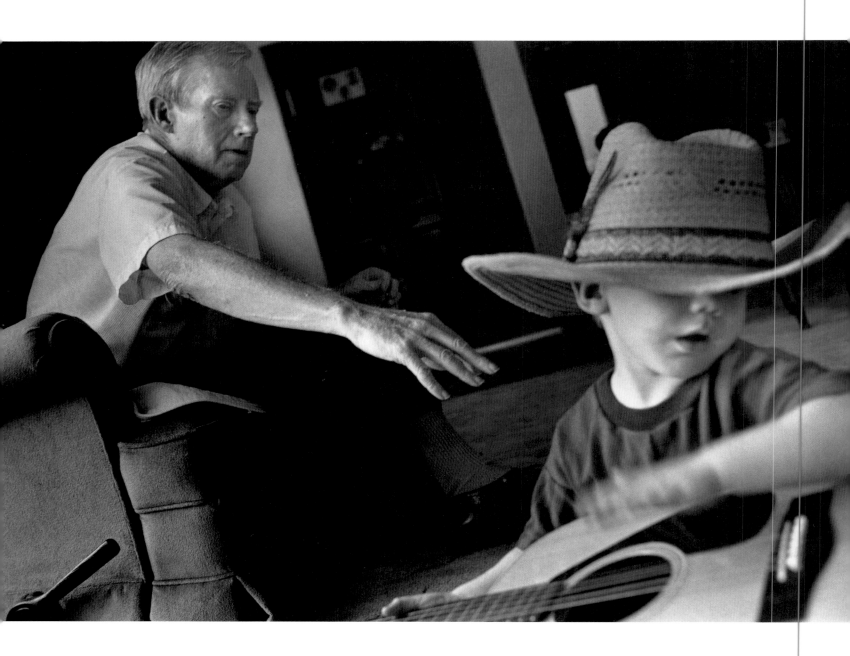

We have music to start off today with—this is Mahler's *Resurrection* Symphony, which I dearly love. And it's a little bit loud, but sometimes, actually, I feel that way. I want to shout. I want to raise some hell. I want to be somebody I'm not.

The only real constant friend I've got is music. I don't have to worry too much—I just turn on the radio and—thank goodness I know how to turn the radio on—and turn it off—I'm not sure about turning it off, but I can turn it on.

17

Sometimes I feel very uneasy about the whole thing, that I should be out making money or I should help people more. I just feel so darn useless at times. I just feel a sense of shame, in a way, for being so unable to do things, and so dense.

Very simply put, we are clumsy, we are forgetful, and our caregivers, of course, understand that, although sometimes I think it must be very hard on the caregivers too, very very hard, because some of us, me for example, can be very very stubborn. We want things to be like they used to be. And we just hate that, the fact that we cannot be what we used to be. It hurts like hell.

And another really crazy thing about Alzheimer's, nobody really wants to talk to you any longer. They're maybe afraid of us, I don't know if that's the trouble or not, I assume it is, but we can assure everybody that we know Alzheimer's is not catching.

I really can't converse very well at all. So that's very limiting. I can't think of things to say before somebody's already said it and they've superseded what I had to say. The words get tangled very easily and I get frustrated when I can't think of a word. Every time I converse with somebody, there's always some word I can't remember. I really cuss when I can't remember a word.

But just keep in mind that everything you can say or do is partial—you're probably never going to get a sentence—a nice clean sentence that says everything you want to say—those sentences are very rare—but they do come once in a while. I just forgot something I was going to say. That, it will be said, I guess, sometime tomorrow. We still believe that there is something ahead, although we know it's going to be diminished. I want to live my life with some sort of dignity, and with some sort of brains left—having brains would be a doggone interesting thing to do.

Every time I have a feeling that I'm losing—losing contact, losing my brains, whatever it is, I panic. I think the really worst thing is you're so restricted, not so much by other people, but you just feel that you are half a person and you so often feel that you are stupid for not remembering things or for not knowing things. Believe me, no matter how much I might be writing on the subject or thinking on the subject, it still just gets my goat—just the knowledge that I've goofed again—I said something wrong or I feel like I did something wrong or that I didn't know what I was saying—that's one of the things—or I forgot—all of these things are just so doggone common they get your goat sometimes.

I'm not going to be one of those who says, "Oh, everything is gone and everything, well I'm dead." Well, you sometimes feel that way. You feel like you're very very restricted. Nobody has restricted you necessarily but the restrictions are very simple things of how far you can walk without getting lost, when you can do something. You always have the feeling it's pretty partial. And you always have the feeling, I know I do a lot of the times, that you just haven't done it right.

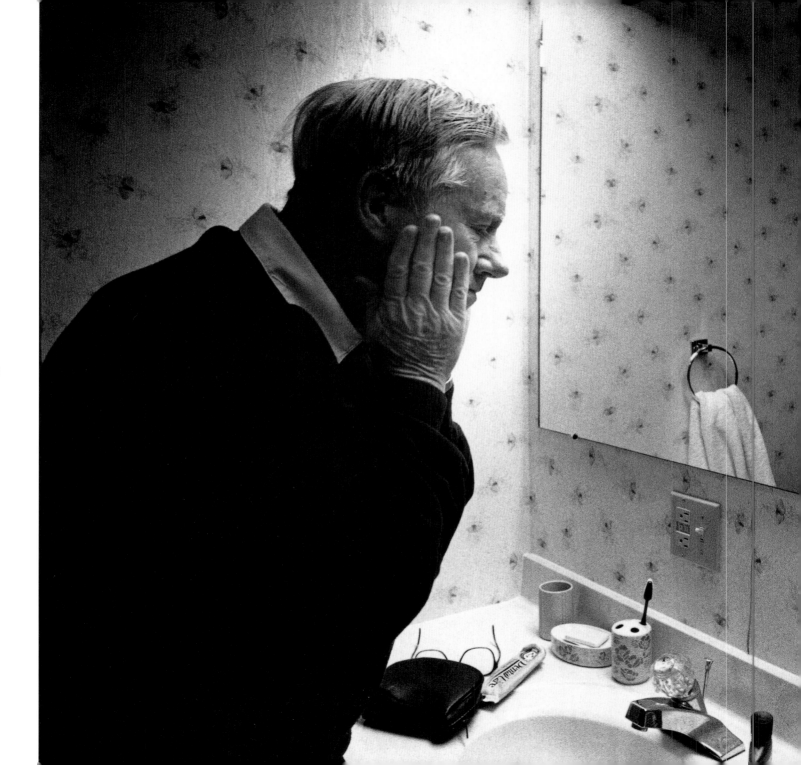

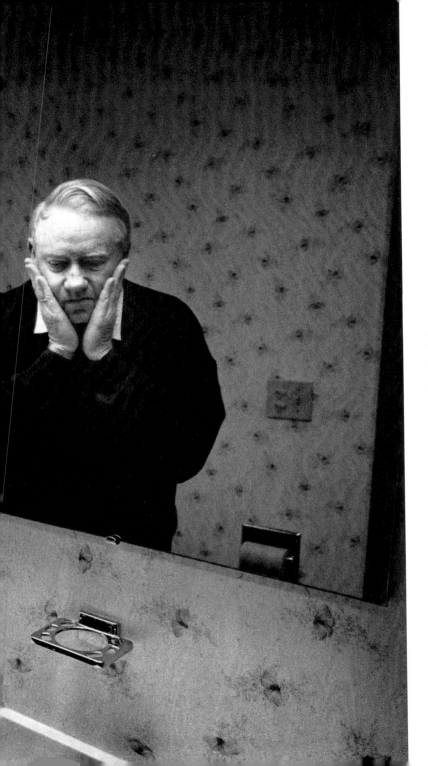

People with Alzheimer's do actually think—they may not think the same sort of things that normal people think, but they do think. They wonder how things happen, why things happen the way they are, and it's a mystery.

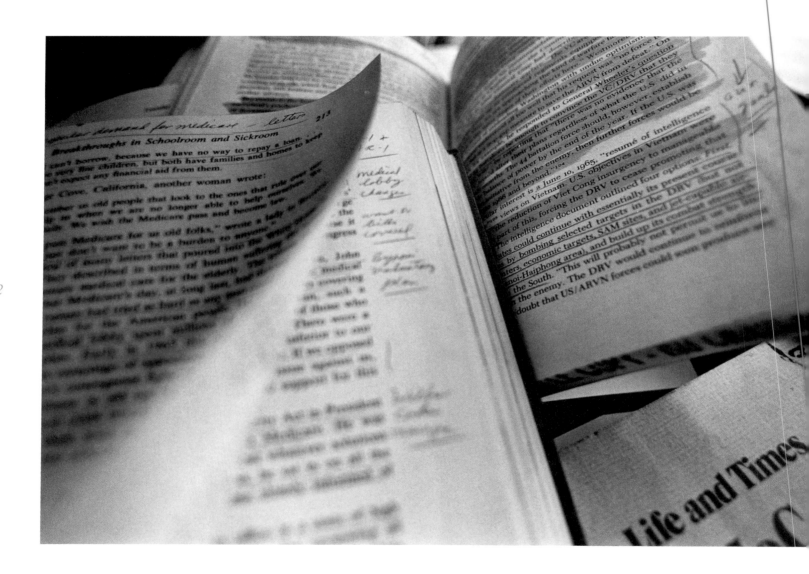

If Alzheimer's had not raised its ugly head, I would just be a professor about to retire from James Madison University. In the teaching profession, when your mind begins to falter, you've had it. Especially something like history. History is something that I really love, even though I can't read anything in history nowadays, which is not interrupted by the fact that I've forgotten all that I was reading.

When Alzheimer's was first diagnosed, I quit my job. I didn't have much choice in that respect. James Madison University can't really function with people who can't function.

Reading's almost impossible. For one thing—things don't stand still. Words don't stand still. It appears to me that it's wavering. I can't pin it down—the words—they can be over yonder and over yonder and I can't catch them.

I couldn't read a book if I had to. I tried very many times to actually read a book, even a small book. But the printed word is something that I find very puzzling. I can see the letters and I can halfway understand what they're all about, but if I try to put the letters in a logical sequence, I'll probably not be able to read.

I can see the words, I can pronounce the words, but they don't seem to mean a whole lot.

I'd like a larger world than I have right now.

Very often I wander around looking for something which I know is very pertinent, but then after a while I forget all about what it was I was looking for. When I'm wandering around, I'm trying to touch base with— anything, actually.

If anything appeared I'd probably enjoy it, or look at it or examine it and wonder how it got there. I feel very foolish when I am wandering around not knowing what I'm doing and I'm not quite always sure how to do any better. It's not easy to figure out what the heck I'm looking for. Once the idea is lost, everything is lost and I have nothing to do but wander around trying to figure out what was it that was so important earlier.

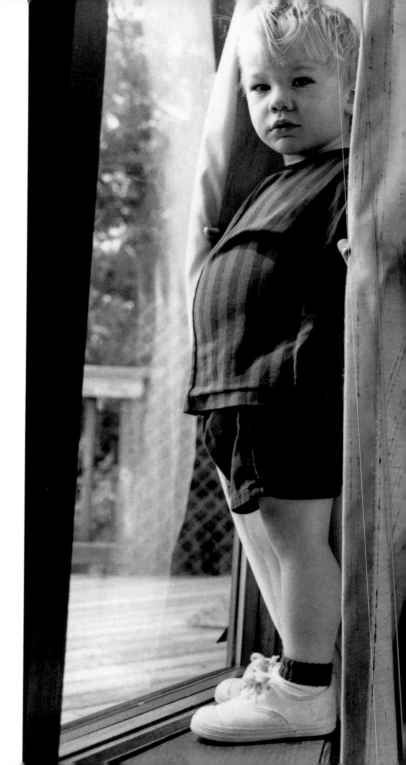

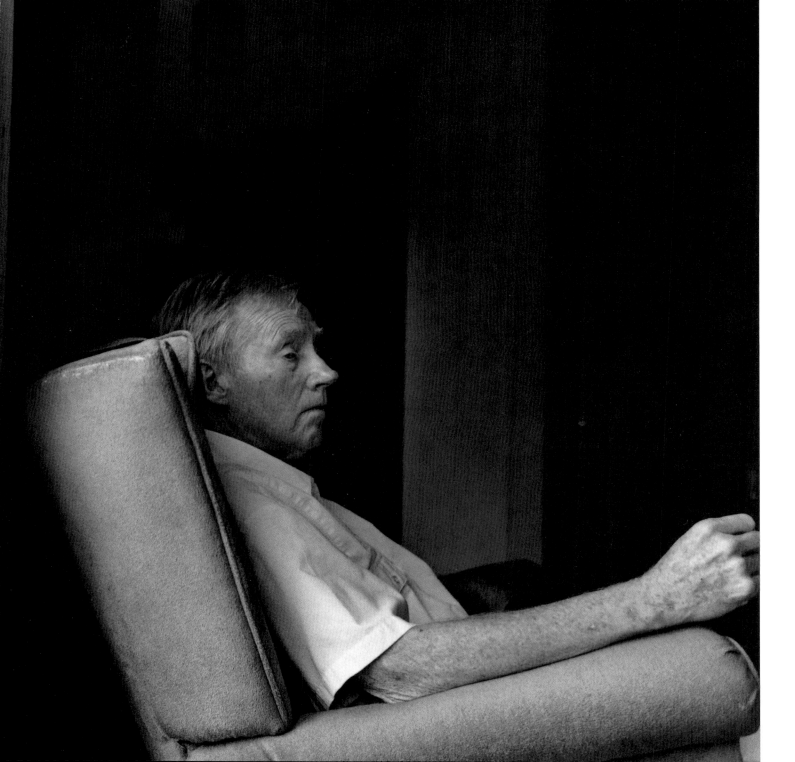

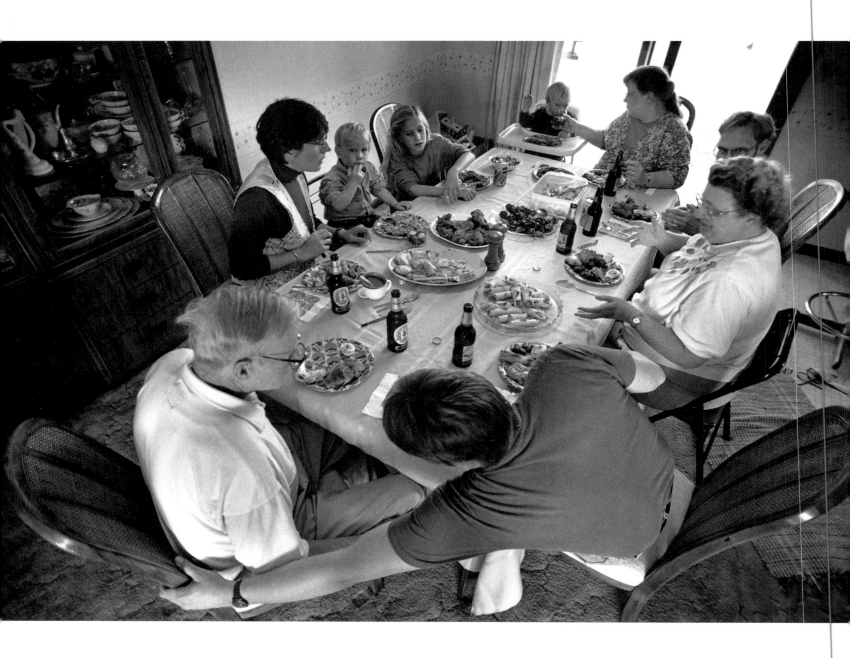

And you have to follow—have to learn to follow—have to learn to be satisfied with what comes to you.

I think the only way to do it is just go with the flow. If you accidentally sit down where people are eating, go ahead and eat. That's my motto: Do as the Romans do. And when Romans do it, if you see Romans doing it, it's all right. As long as they know what they're doing and you know what you're doing, and you're not too far away from somebody who knows what he or she is doing. If you ever get too far away from somebody who knows where they're supposed to be and what they're supposed to be doing, you may well get lost too. So the thing here is—don't get lost.

My wife is trying extra hard to make things tolerable for me—to give me things to do and make me feel good. I really, really do appreciate that. If you're going to get Alzheimer's, by all means, pick out a good caregiver as they call these people, like my wonderful wife, and it's about the best you can do.

I'm afraid of losing contact. She's the only one who really understands me and I'm hard to understand.

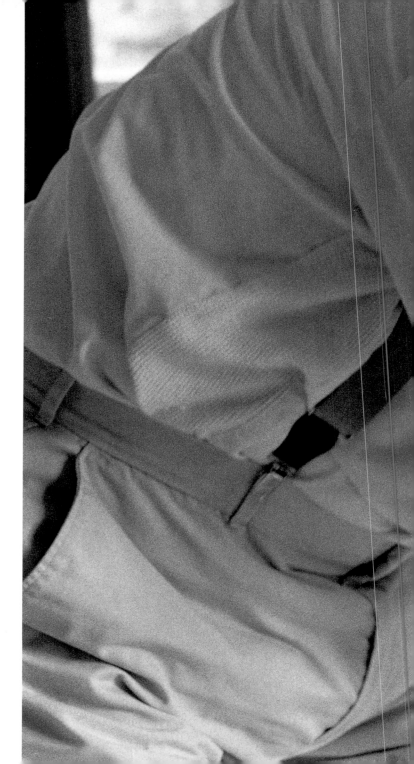

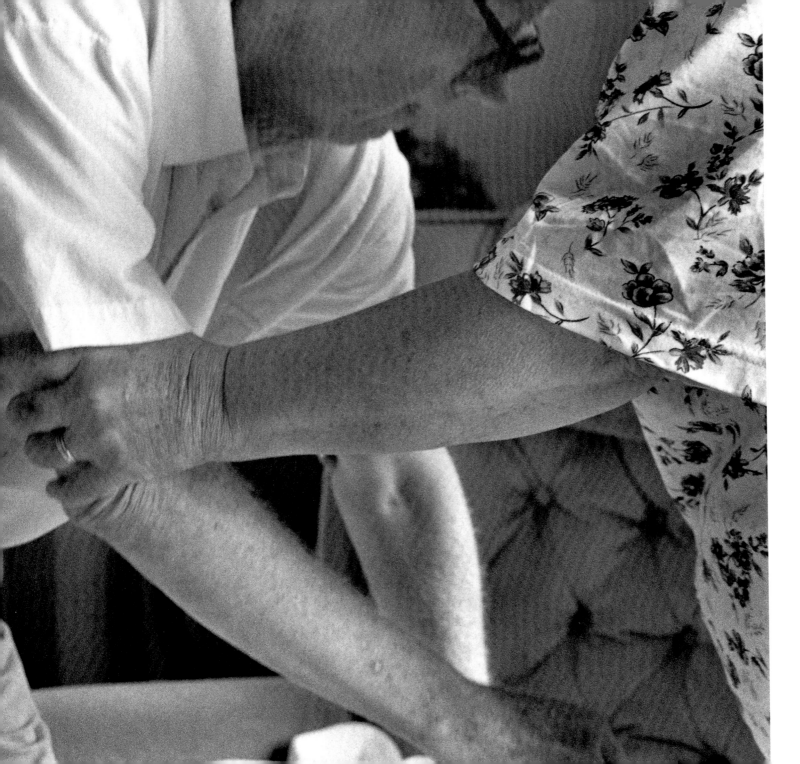

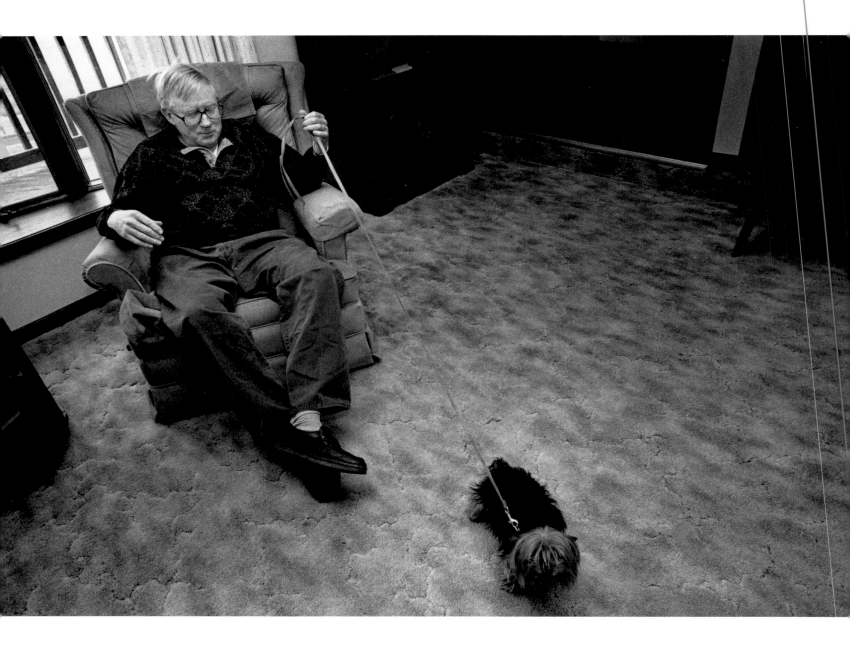

As I've discovered, sometimes even a caregiver might get sick. My wife, who never gets sick, kinda got sick today. And our daughter had gone to sleep—she works at night—which kind of left me on my own lights, and I'm uneasy.

My dog, precious little dog, of course, has to eat once in a while, and my wife was sleeping and I don't know how to open the can of dog food. So the best I could do was to try to dig a hole, make a little perforation and see if I could extend the side of it, and it was something of a panic. The dog has not really been fed yet and I can't possibly wake up my wife, so things are kind of at a standstill right now. My doggie appears to be almost satisfied, but not really. I just hope my wife is not really sick; she's been through a lot trying to take care of me for one thing and our money resources for another thing, and it's just a—kinda crazy.

This was a real, first-rate panic. I opened up the can with a—let's see, what did I use for that—uh, well, whatever came at the moment. I had to find some way to get the doggie some food. But this was one of those things that you're—must get into if you're going to have a life with Alzheimer's. I'm too clumsy, because of the damned Alzheimer's, my feet and legs, oh well, my hands, to do their job, and the best I can do is kind of wiggle them and try to get mad and other silly things. But after tearing up the can, and tearing up a can is a real experience, but maybe my wife, one of these hours, will be feeling better and she can really open the can. Right now, the doggie seems to be in fairly good shape—I am not sure I am.

There's so many things about Alzheimer's that are rather bewildering. Sometimes you can have mood swings that are really awful I think. Sometimes I feel on top of the world, a couple of days ago I did and today I just feel absolutely devastated . . .

Sometimes I might appear to be cocky and sure that everything's all right, that I'm on top of the world. But actually, I'm far from being on top of the world. One day at a time is about the maximum—good days—bad days—bad days—good days—you just never know. This day, my head is all tingly. It just feels very very unpleasant, little needles or something in my head. And I also have a hard time thinking right now—I just can't get organized at all.

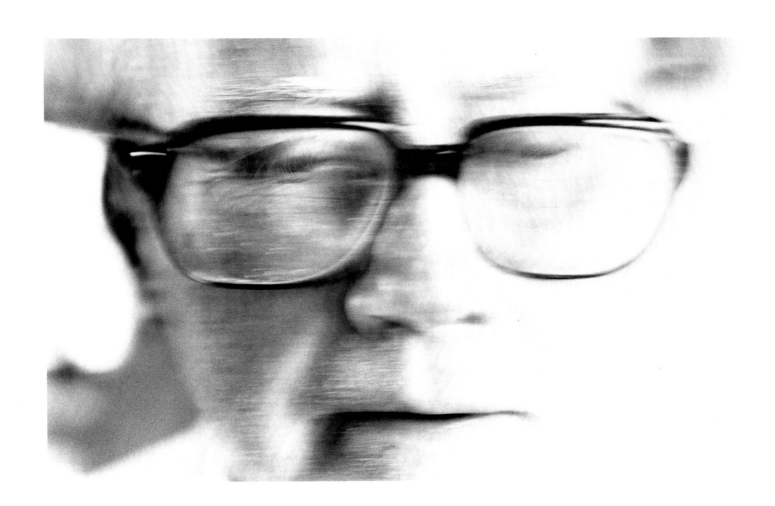

33

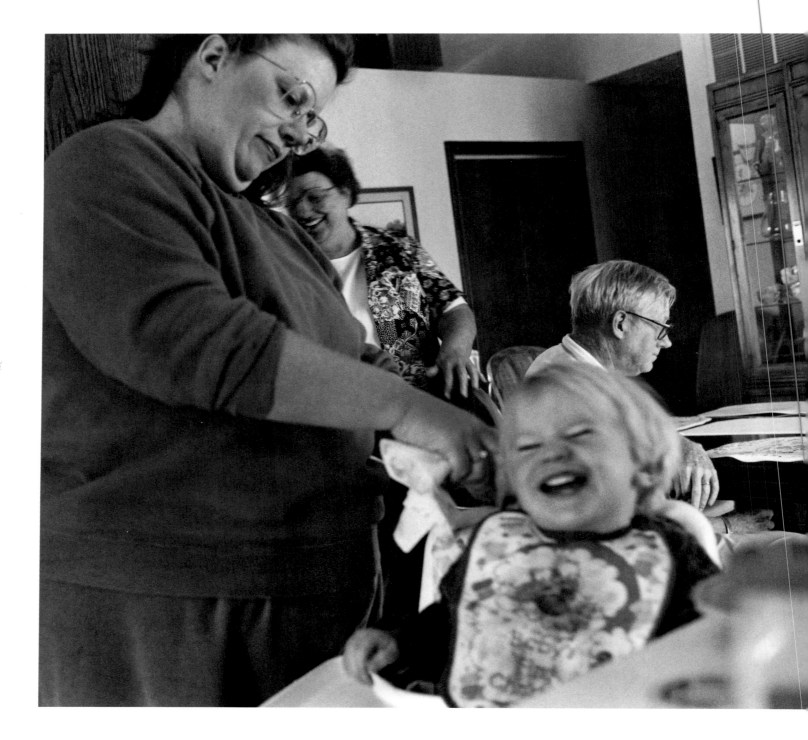

Sometimes I'm jealous of the kids.

I've been thinking about myself. Some time back, we used to be, I hesitate to say the word, "human beings." We worked, we made money, we had kids, and a lot of things we did not like to do and a lot of things we enjoyed. We were part of the economy. We had clubs that we went to, like Kiwanis Club and Food Bank. I was a busy little bee. I was into all sorts of things, things that had to do with charities, or things that had to do with music. Just a lot of things I did back when I was, I was about to say—alive—that may be an exaggeration, but I must say this really is, it's living, it's living halfway.

But one thing is for sure. You never can be, never will be, what you once were. And that's hard to swallow. It certainly was for me. I was very busy in all sorts of things when I was alive, you might say. Then, just gradually, these things became impossible. So we must factor that in, I suppose, something that's going to be with us forever, as long as we live at least. It's either that or die, and dying is something that you have to plan for and want very much. I'm not that much into dying right now—yet.

A lot of things that I don't understand, even after somebody tells me. If I could signal in some way and tell them, oh sure, I heard it, but the ramifications of whatever the heck it was that I heard, I kind of missed.

Being dense is a very big part of Alzheimer's. And forgetting things. Although I'm not as bad as I sometimes am, it comes and goes. It's a very come and go disease. When I make a real blunder, I tend to get defensive about it, a sense of shame for not knowing what I should have known. And for not being able to think things and see things that I saw several years ago when I was a normal person, but everybody by this time knows I'm not a normal person—and I'm quite aware of that.

One of the most interesting things about Alzheimer's is that you're always a little bit behind in your thinking process. You can be thinking a very very essential thought one day, one minute, actually, and somehow you'll lose it. You'll lose what you were trying to say. And the chances are you'll hear it again somewhere but it may not be when you expect it to appear. These thoughts just come very quickly, and go very quickly. And there's not much you can do about it. You could smile about it, I guess.

One of the things, I guess, people like myself with Alzheimer's put up with is the fact that other people have to put up with us. I think the disease does make us kind of irrational. Sometimes it's out of fear and sometimes it's being seemingly left out of things. But it's hard to not be suspicious and I sure hope that nobody holds that against me. I think it's one of the things about Alzheimer's, because we see that other people can work normally and talk normally and have normal experiences and, for some reason, people with Alzheimer's really don't have the—stability I guess you'd have to say, the, I don't know what it is.

But I do think it's bad that we sometimes become almost afraid of ourselves and almost afraid of our caregivers and, of course, our family. But it's awful hard to do sometimes. The feeling of being put on and the feeling of nobody loves us, I think those are perfectly normal feelings. It doesn't mean that you always have to feel that way, but I think for a lot of us the feeling of being cheated, or the feeling of being belittled and somehow made jokes of, I think that's one thing that is among the worst things about Alzheimer's. People like your wife or husband who sacrifice an awful lot, watching us get more and more of this disease, and I guess from their standpoint it is very difficult for them to see us, and vice versa.

The fact of the matter is that the caregivers, usually our family—husband or wife—very often they do things that we are not invited to and you just have to remember, I've got to remember as well as anybody else, that's a normal reaction. We don't really know a lot of things and we misinterpret an awful lot of things and I guess we get to be a damn nuisance ourselves. They get an apology for all of this, but this is something Alzheimer's is going to foist on you— a sense of paranoia.

37

I don't know what to do about it. I guess pulling it out and looking at it for what it really is, is a pretty healthy thing. We know very well that our wives and husbands are not going to try to hurt us, fool us, or in any way put anything over on us. I think probably all of our caregivers, bless their souls and hearts, they do go through a little bit of hell themselves—a lot of it— and a lot of it is because of us.

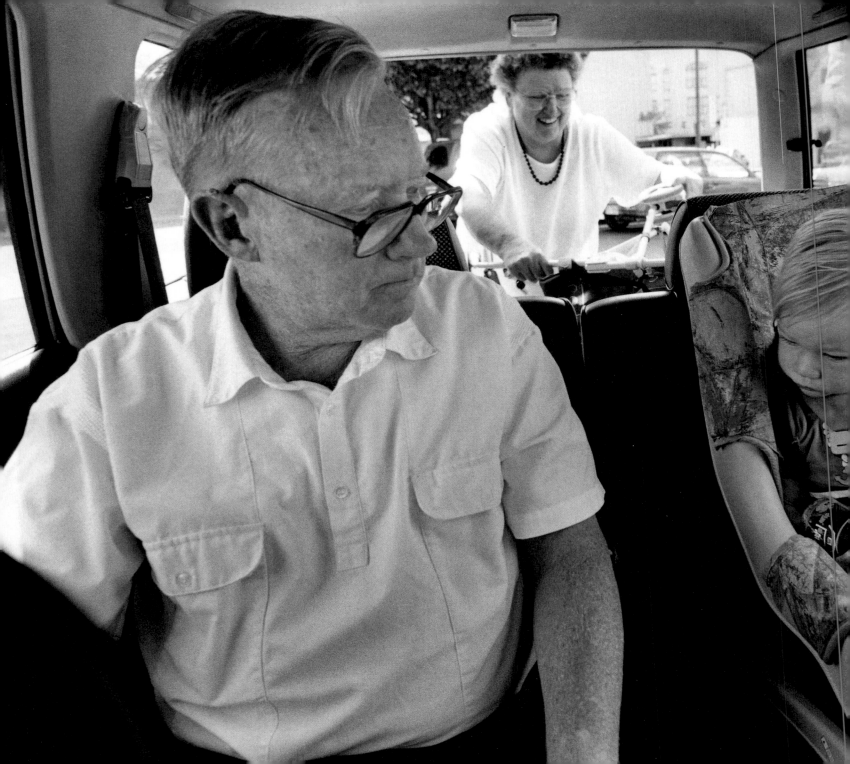

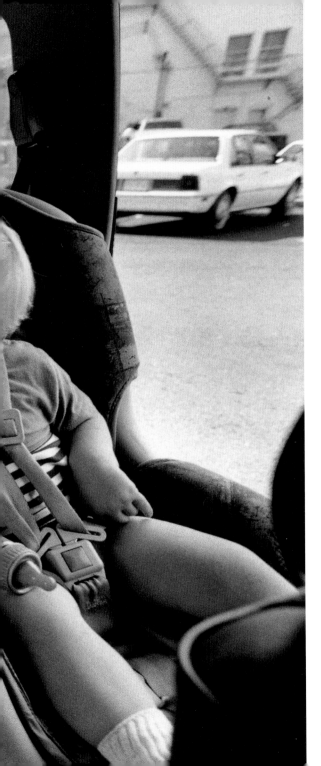

This is a dull life—I grant you. It's a very very dull life. And I guess Alzheimer's patients are urged to go hither and yon, to where people want them to go, because they don't want to leave us at home all the time. Yet, on the one hand we get in the way and on the other hand, we don't really know what's going on most of the time.

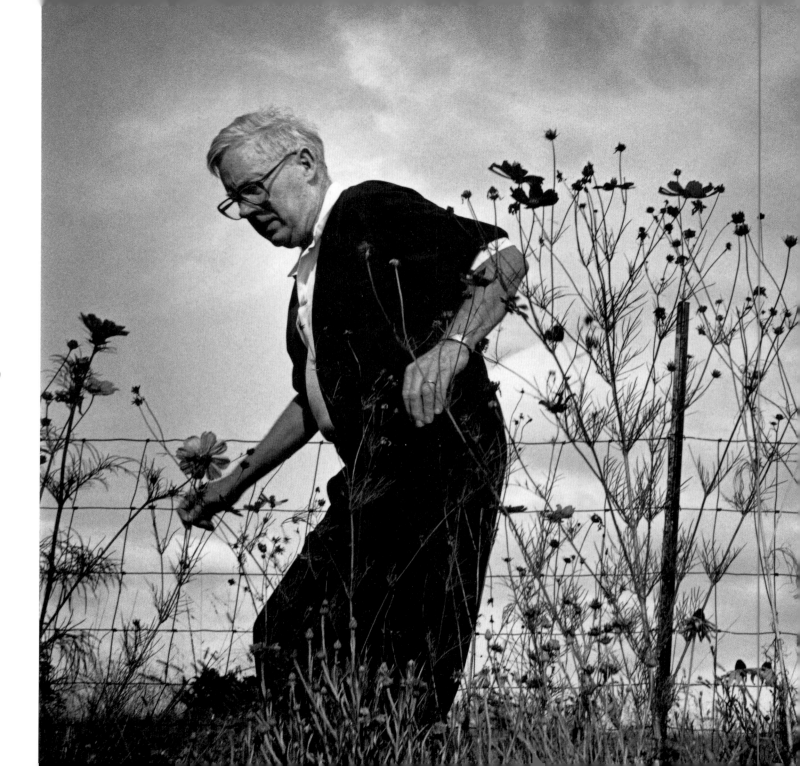

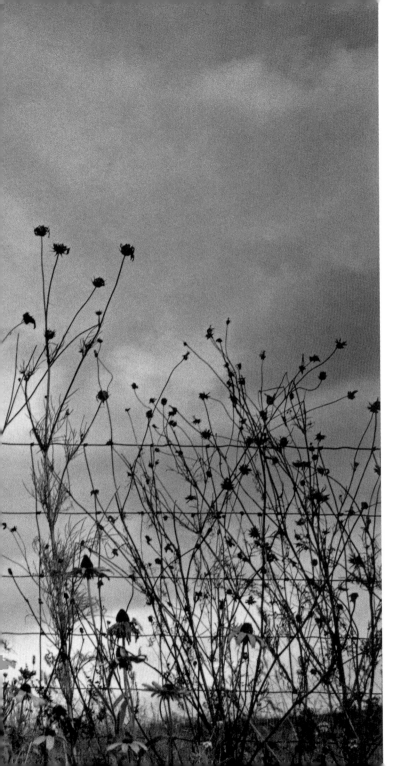

Every day

Is a new day.

I've never seen

This day before

And chances are

I'll never see it again.

Every day is separate.

You don't know

What's going to happen

In any one day.

It's as if every day

You have never seen

Anything before

Like what you're seeing right now.

Every day is absolutely separate

And every minute is separate.

No two minutes

Are anywhere near alike,

Except that you've probably forgotten

Something that you wanted

To remember

In that short time.

Hello, dear audience. I guess since Alzheimer's became obvious, I think I've probably lost something almost every day. Something that I can't find for a long long time and I've forgotten all the configurations of it and I still don't know what the heck it's all about. And anyway, I think anybody with Alzheimer's who doesn't lose something every day, uh, is not a real one, not a real loser.

Today I was just really ready to burst out and do something interesting and fulfilling and all other sorts of things like that, and then I learned that I couldn't find my glasses. And, for what seemed to be eternity, I was running round and round and round trying to find my glasses. Eventually, they showed up. They always do.

Many of us have been on a recycling binge and Alzheimer's has its own variation of this. With Alzheimer's we do forget very rapidly almost anything it's possible to forget. But it can be recycled. I believe that every bit that you hear and see and everything that your brain stores is going to come back to you in one way or another. Ideas do disappear, but once in a while you do find an idea that you'd forgotten before. Sometimes you can reincarnate some of the ideas that you have had.

I've always loved music very very deeply and I find this is a solace. It fills up time and it gives me something to do—listening and ferreting out records that I'm fond of. I think it's a great way to keep time and waste time. And it's also fun. I like classical music, especially Mahler and Richard Strauss, and, of course, the Vienna people.

I've whiled away many many hours listening to music. I can just listen to music and feel that I'm doing something that I just love to do. I can't make music anymore, but I can certainly use it for my own intentions—which are just to be beautiful.

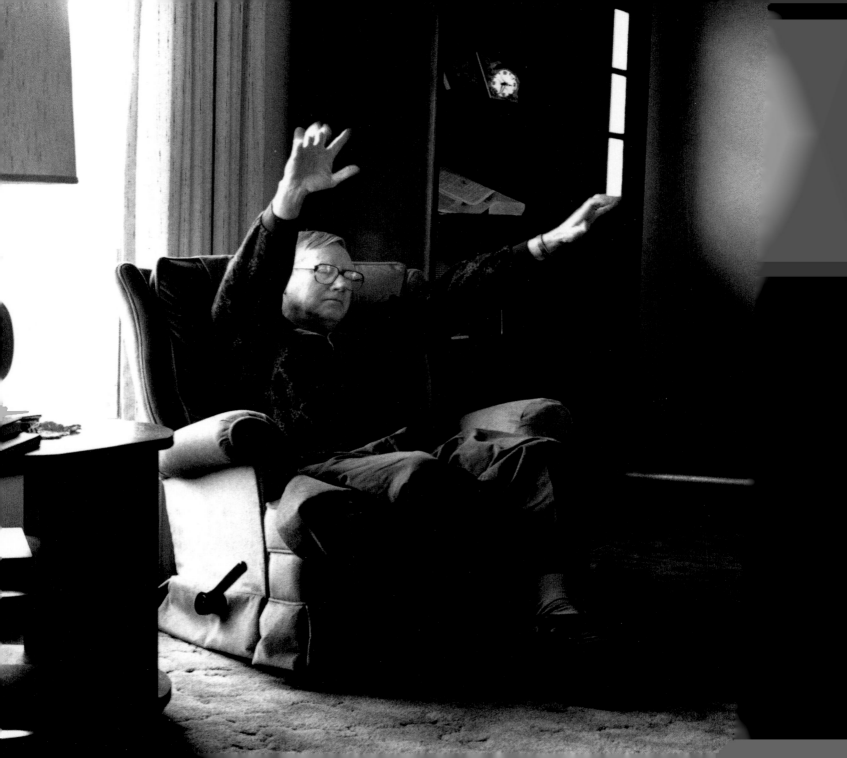

Once again I feel rather old—a little bit over sixty years of age and I'm still reasonably functioning, although I'm—let's call it Level B—which means you're not responsible for anything, you can't remember anything much, but after a while, you get some memory back, and then of course, sometimes you don't. My whole family is here, I guess kind of on and off, and it ought to be real fun and we can celebrate my birthday.

Sixty and sixty-one seem to be, today is sixty-two, my wife tells me, and that's a whole year older than I think it should be, but I guess it's all right. Actually I keep thinking I am hearing different numbers for how old I am—uh—it doesn't make a whole lot of difference— except to people to whom it makes a lot of difference. When you get to these advanced ages, you're not quite so careful about chronicling or looking for dates. The only thing I personally can tell is, it's fairly old, but not really bad old.

For some odd reason, I can't always remember how old I am, and how old I will be in the next day or two. But I guess that's part of the mystery of life. I really don't remember what month I'm living in—it really doesn't make all that much difference.

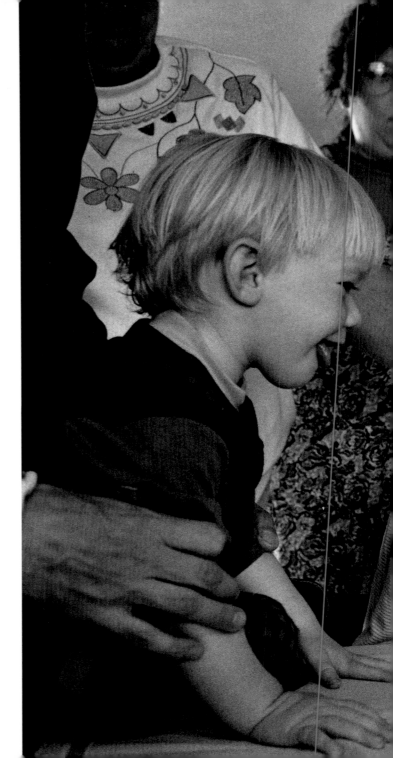

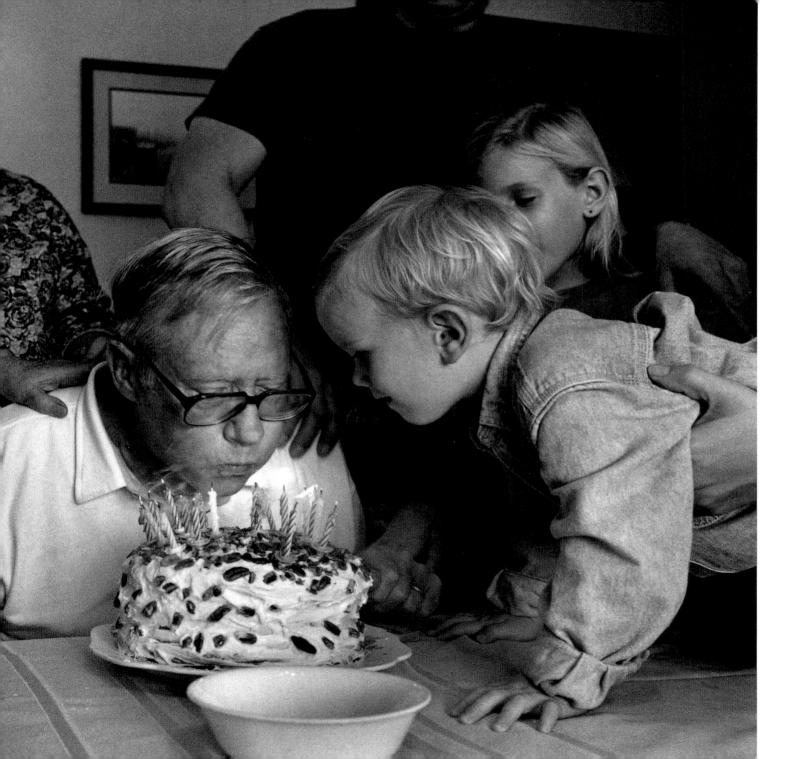

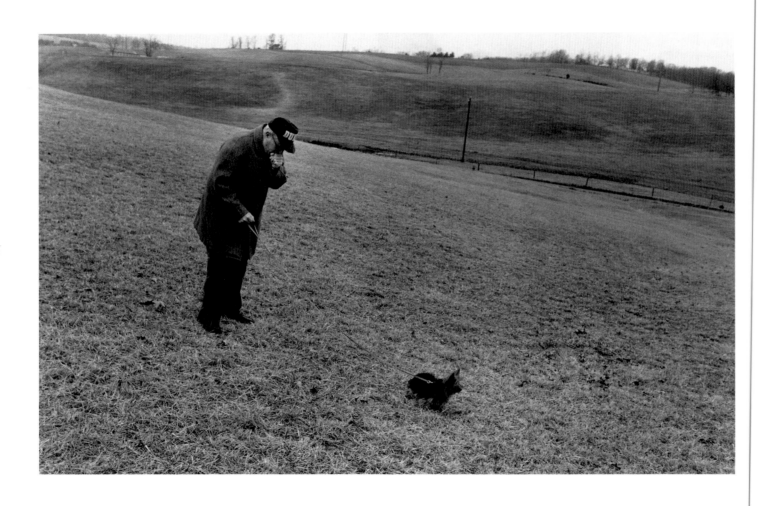

No two days and no two moments are the same. You can't build on experience. You can maybe guess what's going to happen a little while from now—minutes from now, hours from now—we don't know what to expect.

The scariest thing is, I guess, the fact that I have no sense of time. I have not the slightest idea—my brain doesn't—what's ten hours away or what's two hours away.

And if I think that somebody's been, that my wife had been gone a while, I get very antsy. And it may be just a short time that she's been away—it feels like forever.

I feel like it's time long before anybody else feels like it's time. It's just some kind of time warp.

I get really itchy, antsy, whatever you want to call it and it's kind of hard to contain myself. In an emergency the best thing to do is take the dog out for a walk.

Sometimes I kind of wear out my little baby and right now she has been around enough for a while. I normally go out with my little doggie twice a day. That is when she gets her food and assimilates her food and she's ready to get rid of what's left of her food. So I go out twice a day to process my little doggie.

I really think that a dog is a great asset to somebody with Alzheimer's. One reason is that they are dumb, they're stupid, they don't know how to do much—but the one thing that they do know is what the master says. I mean that dog knows things about me before I know them myself. She's not exactly a guide dog, that's for doggone sure, she's not a very useful dog, not a working dog—she's just loyal.

There's a lot of things that happen when I'm walking the dog. This morning—it was rather embarrassing—to be living in Harrisonburg, Virginia, now for a long long time—many many years—we've been living in the same place for a long long time, and I still have trouble knowing where things are.

Uni and myself were walking and a lady drove up and asked about the community recreation center. A lot of fun ensued, 'cause I sort of knew where it was and it's not very far from the house. But I got all flustered and she figured I didn't know what the hell I was talking about. In fact, I didn't know what to say. I was kind of stunned by the whole thing, and she drove away.

I've been around the recreation center endless times and I know theoretically where it is and how far it is from home. The recreation center is the tallest and roundest place around, but somehow or another, I just couldn't see it—to figure out what to do with her.

This recreation center thing just took everything and kind of jelled it into one little piece. I've been living around here for years and years and years, and I cannot tell anybody how to go three blocks and go to the recreation center. And I kind of doubt if I ever will be able to.

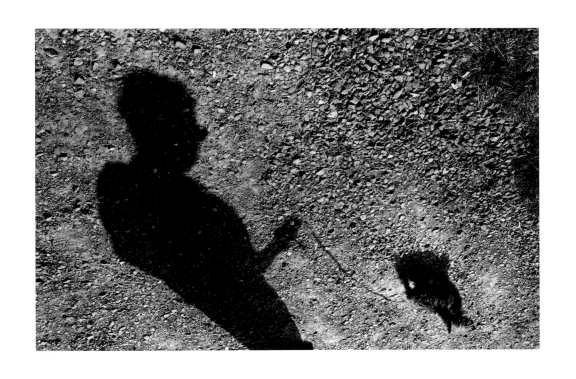

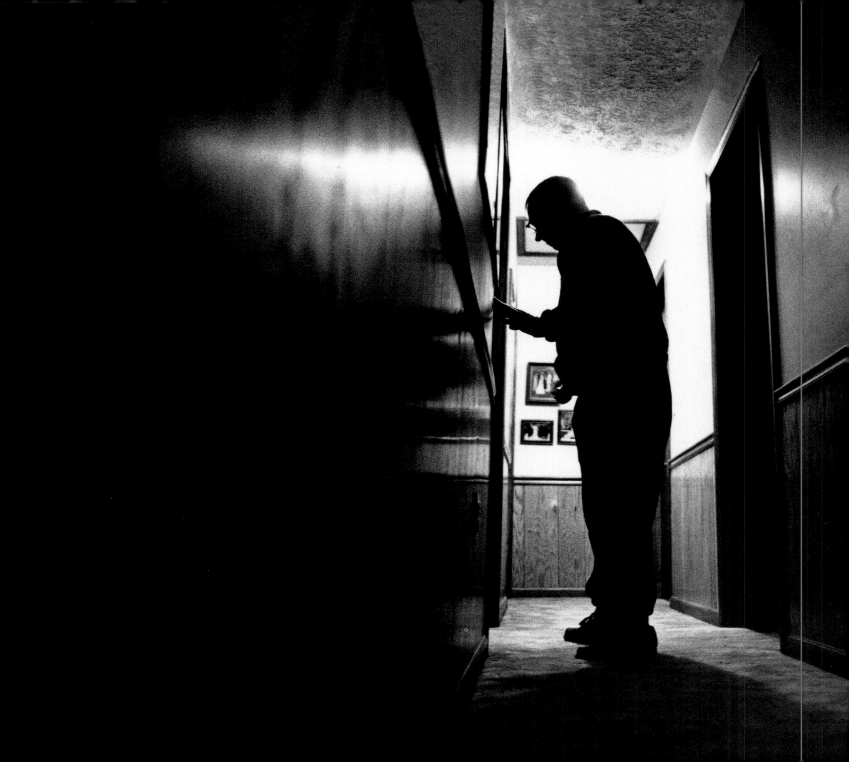

The things that you see and things that you experience in the dark, to me are almost life threatening.

And the dark is a time when you don't see things very well. In the dark you might be just totally lost. That's happened to me before and I wouldn't dare venture out at night by myself. I just can't prefigure things well enough to know what they might be, what the shapes are. So I stay away from that, stay away from the dark as much as I can.

51

I think I've neglected something very important about the family of the caregiver—caregivers. What if somebody, let's say the children, have a tragedy of some sort and they have people like myself who don't have enough brains to figure out what to do?

I wouldn't know how to handle the situation, in fact, there's no way to handle the situation. We really don't know what the heck we're doing. My daughter today had a very very bad situation, how well she is we don't know. She's very sick and we're very much concerned about her and she's at the hospital and I'm at the house. Of course, I'm by myself and I don't have any idea what's going on except that I don't believe there's a whole lots that's favorable for Jackie.

We are parts of families most of us—we don't have a huge family—we do stick together pretty well. We've so far not had any situation of this sort, but this one really does appear to be serious and right now the medical people and us are all unable to figure out what's going on. And I'm in the house and they're in the hospital, and I wouldn't know how to get to the hospital myself if I had to. It's one of those things.

So, the truth is I'd be helpless whether I was where she is or at home where I am. But the fact is I'm home by myself—don't know anything.

The daughter who is now sick is the one who is— was—putting together my memoirs and I can only say,

very selfishly, I hope she's able to come back and beat 'em all, but one of the things we have to do is wait and see—and hope.

So the dog and I are waiting to know what is going on with our daughter. So far I think I've given the impression that it's just the caregiver and myself, but in the real world there are others involved.

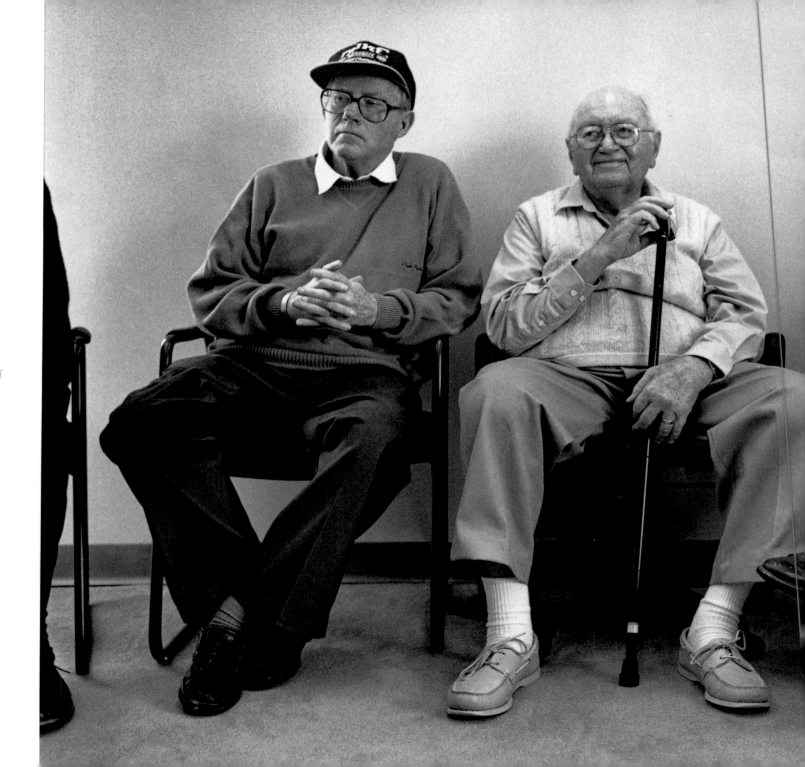

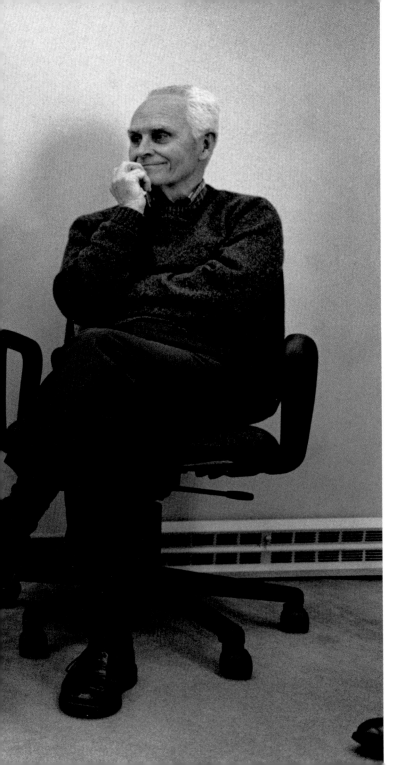

I've been at this Alzheimer's thing quite a while now. I don't enjoy Alzheimer's. I'll say that for you, for me— but there's something in it that I feel rather at home with people with Alzheimer's.

I think one of the worst things about Alzheimer's is you're so alone with it. Nobody around you really knows what's going on. And half the time, most of the time, we don't know what's going on ourselves. I would like some exchange of views, exchange of experiences, and I think for me at least, this is a very important part of life . . .

It would be interesting for Alzheimer's patients to correspond with one another, not necessarily to learn very much, but to, just to see what other people are thinking. Well, if you're like me, I'm not sure you're thinking a whole lot, but you have a lot of feelings, I must say a heck of a lot of feelings. Everything we do is just full of feelings.

I don't know about the wisdom of having a get-together of Alzheimer's patients. It'd be a real gasser, I'm sure, but I don't know if it would be worth anything. But I really would sincerely like to share my—our—experiences and our feelings, and what I'm trying to do in this series of talks, if that's what you want to call it, these are straight from the victim's own words and whatever I say is sincere. Even though maybe maybe someday I'll make some sense.

We do have feelings and we do have some kind of knowledge. It may not be very profound, but nevertheless I think we do have experiences which might be worthwhile, especially to anybody who had any reason at all in this world to want to know a little bit about Alzheimer's. I do suspect that we do know more than we seem to know because it gets so hard to express what we know.

We can't turn the clock back and we can't turn a lot of things back, but maybe we can get a feeling of stasis—we do exist and we do have feelings, we do have notions. To some degree, we can be just like any other people, although we do forget more and we lose more. We really do want to be like human beings, we have so many fears, the fear of forgetting things—the fear of tripping over something—our speech is not too clear sometimes and our feelings are hard to sort out many many times. I'd just like to know from anecdotal experiences that people with Alzheimer's have had, to what degree are they clumsy, to what degree do they very quickly forget things, and to what degree they can make themselves useful. I try to put the dishes on the table as much as possible and do as many chores as I possibly can do. And my wife lets me do that, thank goodness. You need to have something that you can do even though the fact is there are not too many things you can safely get into.

I don't go to movie theaters any longer—it seems to be too stifling and that's another little thing—just like I've been talking about— Are most people with Alzheimer's afraid of the dark? Are they afraid to be alone? Do they like to go out to the movie houses? I much prefer seeing the movies at home. Mainly because I've got claustrophobia. Do most people with Alzheimer's have claustrophobia? I've got lots of questions. And I have so very few answers.

Claustrophobia is not just being in a small room, it's being anyplace where you can't move around. And, of course, another thing about it is, if you're like me, you stumble very easily. And I don't like for people to see me stumble.

I really want to find out from other people what they have experienced. As for myself, I must admit, I don't know very much. In my little diary here, I'm really giving all I've got. If we see somebody who has Alzheimer's, who might have Alzheimer's, or somebody we know is having problems, perhaps we can help. We can't give them medical help. We can to some degree, I hope, encourage people who have Alzheimer's to not be ashamed and not be any more, you might say mind-paralyzed, than they are . . .

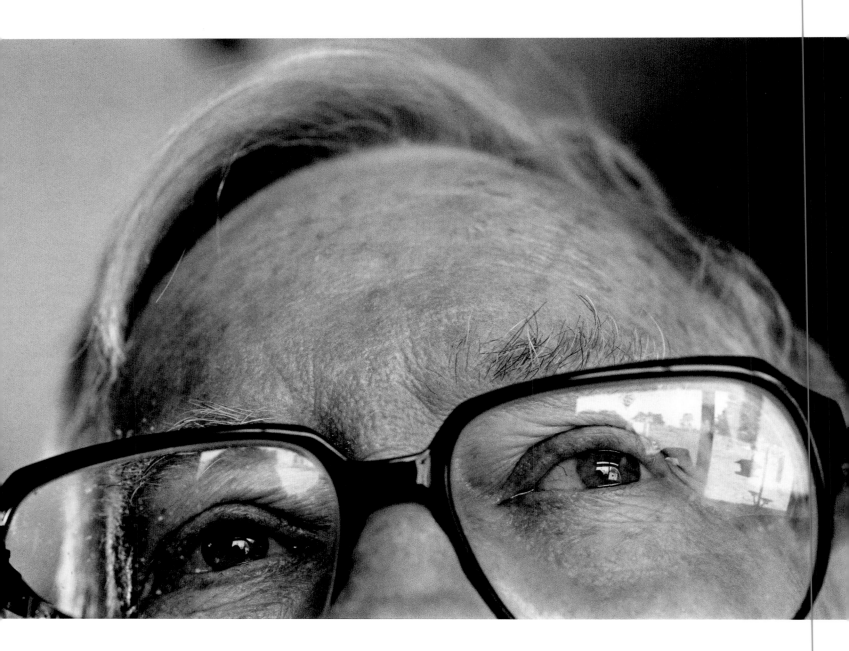

I'm not really sure Alzheimer's is a killer, in the usual sense of the word, it's a maimer. I'm sure, a maimer of—what did I say?—certainly a killer of people's thoughts.

I'm not sure that Alzheimer's kills as such, it certainly does kill the brain, which really sincerely is a whole lot worse than just dying.

Sometimes there is a feeling of guilt for having Alzheimer's. I should have known better. Something should have been different. Maybe I'm no damn good. You're worthless, you can't hack it.

I've thoroughly enjoyed being a guinea pig. Every couple of months, it seems like, I get stuck with several needles to get some blood flowing and they send the blood off to the laboratory in—someplace in the far West—and they do whatever they have to do . . . Durham is a second home. It's where you have people who know what it's about and they're willing to work with you and they test us every time we go there to see how we've improved—or not improved, and just in general to do all they can to keep you going.

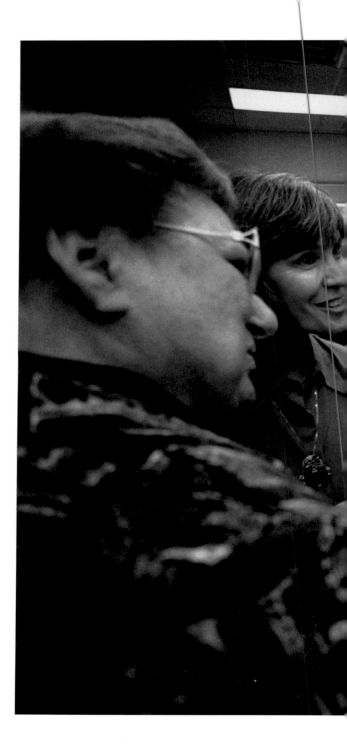

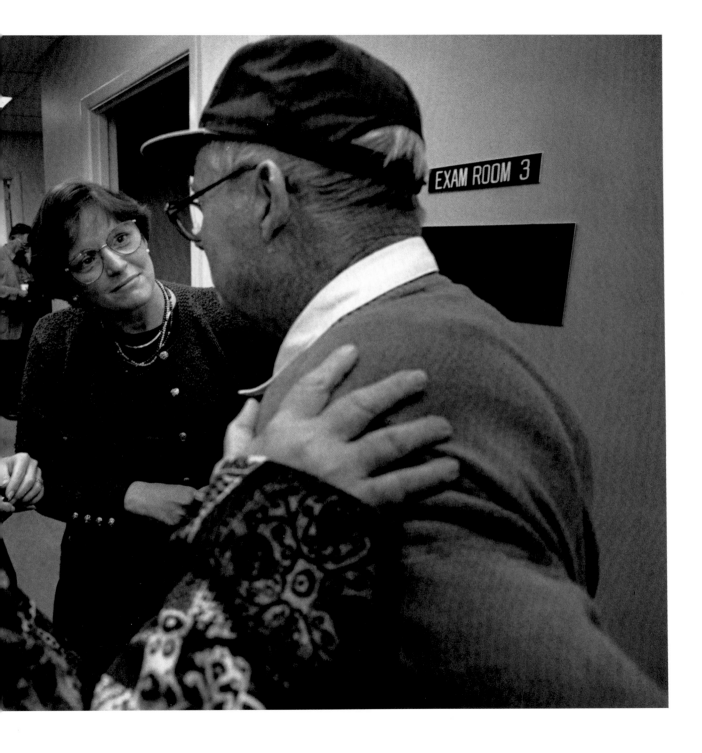

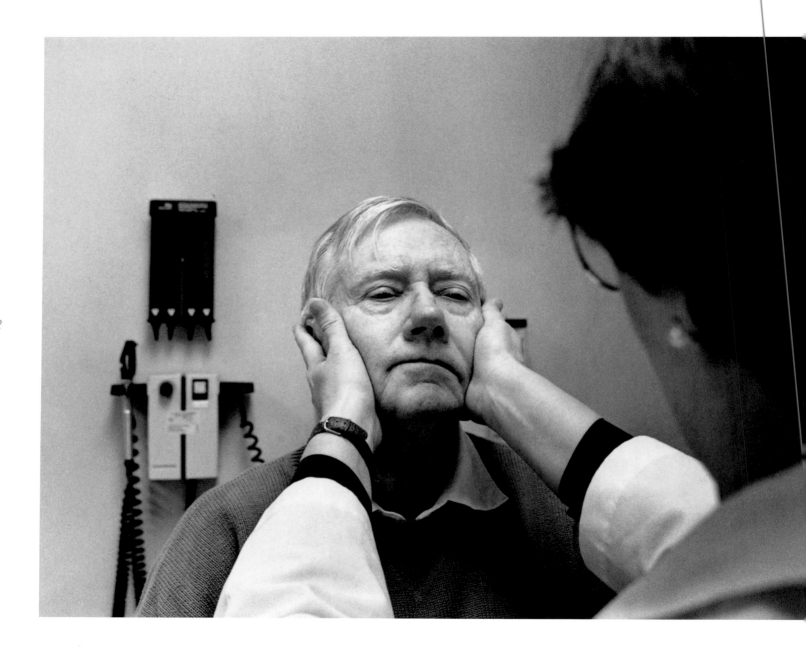

The lady who is in charge of this, let's see, what is her, a big boo-boo here, she's been in charge of it since I've been going there and she is one of the nicest people in the whole world. She's very devoted to helping Alzheimer's people . . . Sarah, yeah . . . she just got remarried.

We've had another one of our experiences in Durham concerning the disease and I'm going to be in some —a lot of tests—one reason being I have the most beautiful brain in the world, I guess, in a sense—it's a great honor to have something like that 'cause I'm probably the best diagnosed person Alzheimer's has ever had, so they kind of measure me for norms, I guess . . . They bring me back to Durham almost all the time— whenever they need whatever it is, some of my blood or something else, and it's kind of fun. I feel like I'm

doing something not only interesting but I think something that's needed.

I feel like something of a pioneer, and sometimes they will probably draw a whole bunch of blood, but as one of the very few absolutely verified Alzheimer's people—it has been shown by biopsy—that's the best thing you can find in purity, so with the biopsy you can be absolutely sure I am pure, no strings attached. I'll be giving blood again I'm sure.

And when I get to Durham and I have something I like to do, I'm kind of on a high. It's something that I can do that not everybody can do, and it makes me feel very good about this. It makes me feel like I'm not going to just rot in my old age, helpless and stupid.

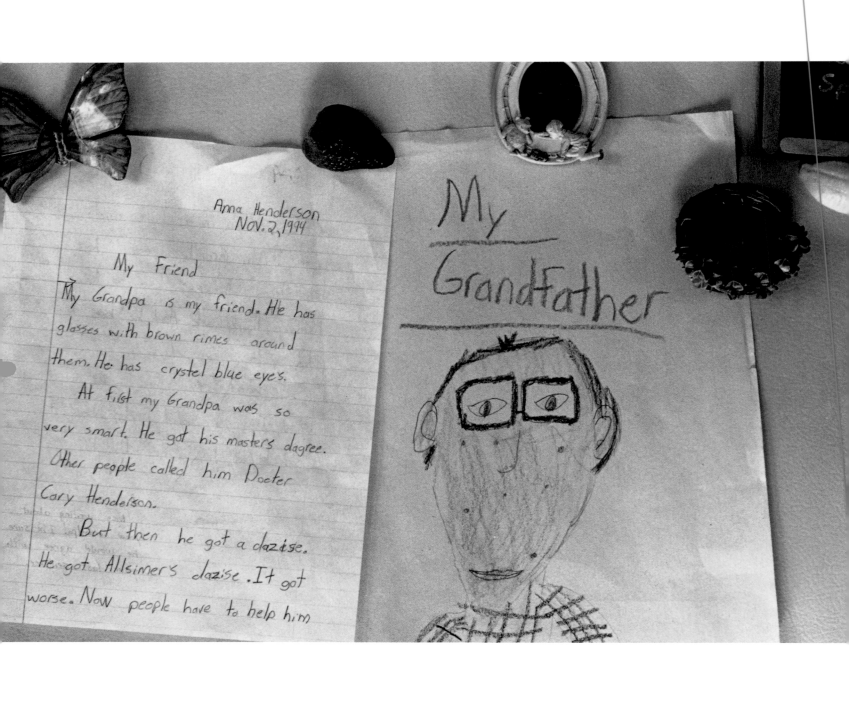

Anna Henderson
Nov. 2, 1994

My Friend

My Grandpa is my friend. He has
glasses with brown rimes around
them. He has crystel blue eyes.

At first my Grandpa was so
very smart. He got his masters dagree.
Other people called him Docter
Cary Henderson.

But then he got a dazise.
He got Allsimer's dazise. It got
worse. Now people have to help him

My
Grandfather

One of the things about this is—it's in the family and the family has not only me and my wife, but we have our children and the children have their spouses. In other words, this whole thing about Alzheimer's is not just about two people, it's about a whole mess of people. Not only our families but our extended families and their friends. It gets very very involved. But that's the way life is supposed to be.

I think that is the one thing that is the most difficult about Alzheimer's—is loving, continuously and without qualms, without holding anything back—it's a matter of trust. I think probably, though, that anybody who is a caregiver to an Alzheimer's patient, their patience is just going to be continually bothered.

But I think love is the key to all this stuff and love is something that my wife certainly has given to me and the family has too and there's nothing that I can see to complain about.

There are times when I feel just terribly sorry for myself. And I would think that would be something Alzheimer's people normally have. Paranoia is with us. I mean it's not going to go away. But even though we do have a good dose of paranoia, we understand that people still love us—our kids and our wives and husbands. They do, honest to goodness, love us, but there are times, and I mean lots of times, where our family and friends really don't know how to take us.

Every once in a while, I will talk to my wife, talk to my daughter, to my son, and an hour later I will say something that makes it very obvious that I haven't remembered a thing that they said. Of course I know that, but it sometimes annoys them.

It mainly bugs my wife—I forget these things that are so important to her. In a way, I guess, they're important to me too, but I don't remember when they are.

I haven't done a whole lot today except think about Christmas. The family has done really the best they can—the love has been quite obvious—that they all want me to have a good Christmas. I'd love for them to have a great Christmas.

And, you know, the doggonest things do occur, like I was asking my wife, "Did I get a present for Jackie?"

Did I get a present for—well, anybody? I couldn't really tell you what present I gave anybody. I'm pretty sure I gave everybody something, but I can't recall what it was and it's kind of embarrassing. It's supposed to keep you in suspense, and everything you see is a revelation that you've not quite seen before.

We've finished with Christmas and New Year's and some time with our kinfolks. Sons and mothers, and everybody else you can think of, seemed to have been here this last few weeks. We're very glad, of course, to know all these people and to know they love us but there's one little thing that somebody in my predicament can probably understand, whenever there's a gathering of people, it seems, at least in my mind, to be a lot of confusion. I just feel the need for quiet.

I can only think of one thing at a time. And large gatherings, whatever they may be, are very very hard to understand.

But I think the factor I've been talking about most recently—the calms. I could remember a lot better if there's not much going on. I can think better. If there's anybody else in the room, it seems like—more than just one person—I do sort of lose my grip.

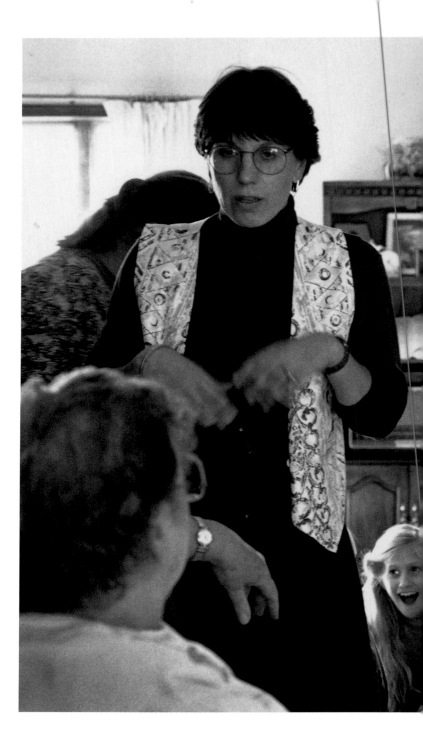

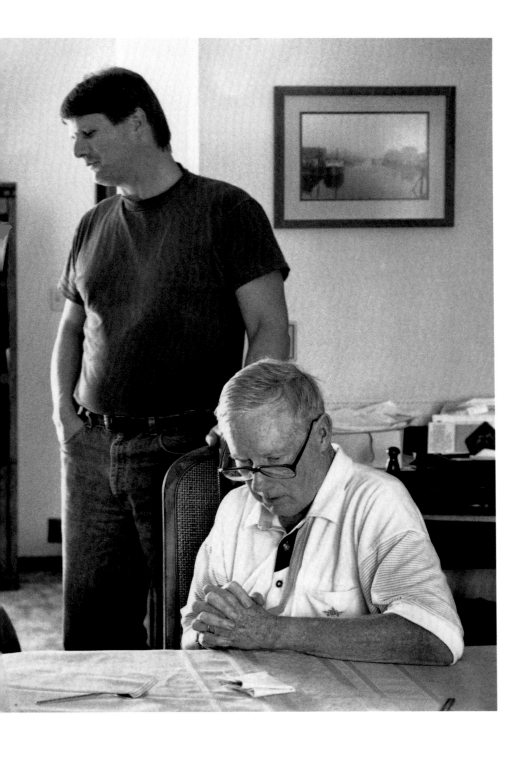

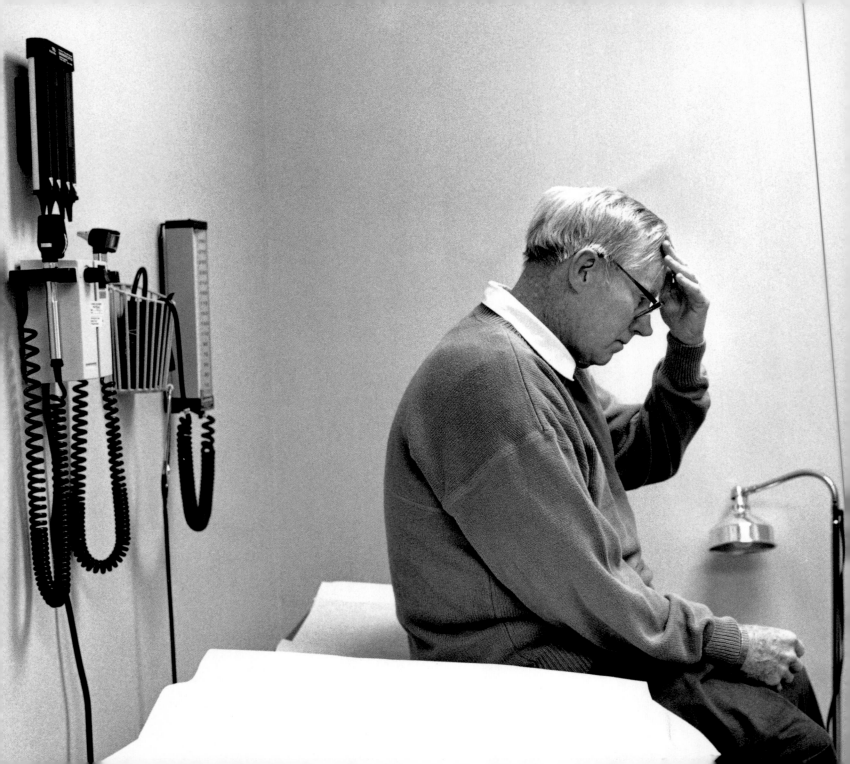

I really sincerely believe that if somebody wants to go ahead and die from Alzheimer's, if life has become that bad for them, I think anybody who can quietly assist them to die, I think, would be a boon.

This Dr. Kevorkian, this doctor way up North who helped people to kill themselves—I think he did the right thing. Apparently all of these people had wanted to die, and had a very very good reason for it.

When your mind is dead or dying and there's no recourse, and the best you can do is spend the rest of your life in pure stupidity and unknowing stupidity . . . I think that is one of the biggest travesties of what sometimes is called medicine that we have ever heard of. It seems like fairly commonly we do read about people who die from Alzheimer's, but we can also speculate about people with Alzheimer's who—they're ready to die. I would think it's just overwhelming them to the point where there's no place to go, no place to hide.

My wife is out now trying to take care of her mother who is in a nursing home, and God, I hope I never get in one of those.

I can just see myself in a nursing home, and God, I hate the idea. I just hope my brain can keep up until I'm dead . . . things like that are very scary . . .

Right now my daughter is upstairs trying to sleep after working all night, and of course my wife is at Oak Lea [nursing home] with her mother, trying to see if her mother wants to go to the mall and if she's able to go to the mall—does she know where the mall is—another question. Actually, I couldn't find the mall either if I tried to. Fortunately, somebody can always drive me there or any other place but that's a real hassle.

My biggest fear is going into a nursing home.

I did stop going to church—the biggest reason—well, there were two reasons—one of which I am not really enamored of a God who creates something like Alzheimer's and the second is I'm afraid of tripping.

Sometimes we miss being important—miss being needed.

Sometimes I just get overloaded with things I think ought to be thought. I feel so much—I guess you might say, in the way. I feel sometimes very much in the way. Someone with Alzheimer's I don't believe can participate fully—sometimes I think I'm doing a pretty good job of it and other days I'm totally at a loss. Confusion reigns. And I would guess it's pretty common that somebody with Alzheimer's really can't cope with more than one thing at a time. And that one thing at a time has to be reasonably easy to understand.

Alzheimer's is a lot of stress, mainly because you know what you have been earlier and you know very well you're not that good now and it's real hard to reconcile. There are times when I've felt like destroying things— sometimes I want to cuss; actually I do some cussing out of frustration. It's a whole lot better, though, if things are quiet and uncomplicated.

I guess what I'm getting to is that we are very second-class citizens in the real sense of the word. We do need to be taken care of. I've learned pretty much the parameters of my life—how far I can go and what I can expect to do and I can live with it—I think. I'm an onlooker to life now, not a participant. An onlooker and philosopher.

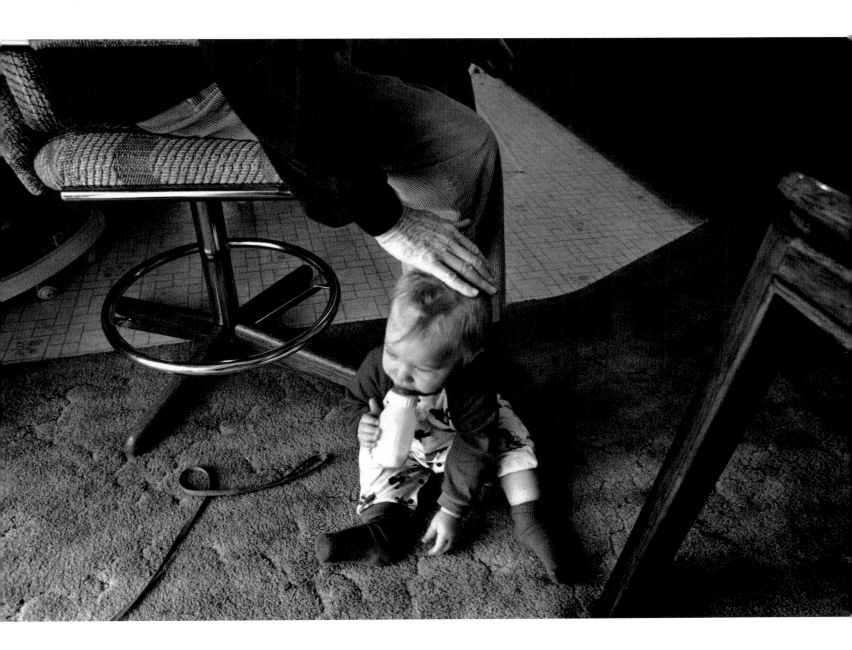

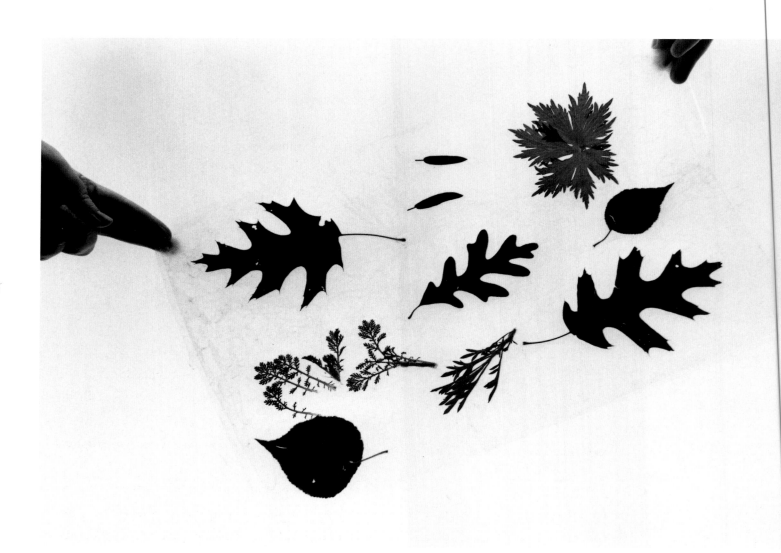

I don't think I'm trapped any longer, like I did at first, and I feel like I can cope with it . . . It's kinda hard though.

Somehow I learned to cope with it, mainly through—first of all, you know you're going to screw up a good many times, so just don't let it bother you. There'll be another time to screw up, and there might be a few times when things go right . . .

When I was first diagnosed, she and I were just absolutely sure that everything was over, that life was just simply going to pot. It's difficult, I think, for somebody with Alzheimer's to not just give up and say, the hell with it. I periodically do that, but then again, there are some things that I really enjoy.

I still pick up leaves, probably the same ones I had before. I love the fall colors. I pick 'em up anyhow, whether I have them or not. Every year it seems like they're prettier and prettier. I appreciate them a lot more now than I did a few years ago.

When I can't do the big things, I can do the little things. Things are a lot more precious than they were. I go ape on the leaves—I collect them whether I have them or

not. I usually have all of them, but I have to carry them home on the chance I don't have one of them.

One of the things which my wife started which I've been really fascinated with is—well, you might call it a bird sanctuary. She puts out feed for the birds and they really seem to enjoy it. It's something really interesting to watch—how many different birds we can get. It's awful hard to say how many there were because they—because they do fly away—they fly back—they fly away. They're kind of unstable.

But we really do enjoy seeing our cardinals and other birds. The cardinals of course are the most spectacular. We have a whole bevy of smaller birds—wrens and goodness knows what else—and just watching them at the bird feeder I think is a fascinating endeavor. I can watch the birds for quite a while—watch them fly in and fly out—which of course is what birds do. And you can hear the coo—coo—coo of the whippoorwill.

The great thing about birds is they don't stay in one place very long. Up and down, up and down, sideways, and everything else. That's probably the most fun thing about birds is the fact—now you see 'em and now you don't.

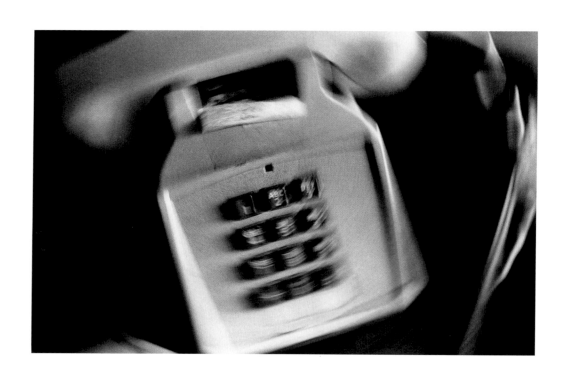

The phone. That's the most frustrating thing on earth. I get nervous trying to use the phone. I get tongue-tied. I can't figure out what the heck I'm doing. If I am the only one at home, it's trouble. I just can't hack it. Even if people eventually hang up—even if they're important people we'd like to talk to, I still can't do it. When they hear that I'm fumbling for words, for a long time, they usually give up.

Speed is absolutely impossible—just forget about speed—we're not going to be fast remembering things and knowing things and doing things.

When someone wants me to hurry up, I can't hurry up—there's no way to hurry up. The hurrier I get, the behinder I go, and I think that's pretty much for anybody with Alzheimer's. We can't be rushed because we get so doggone confused we don't know what we're rushing about.

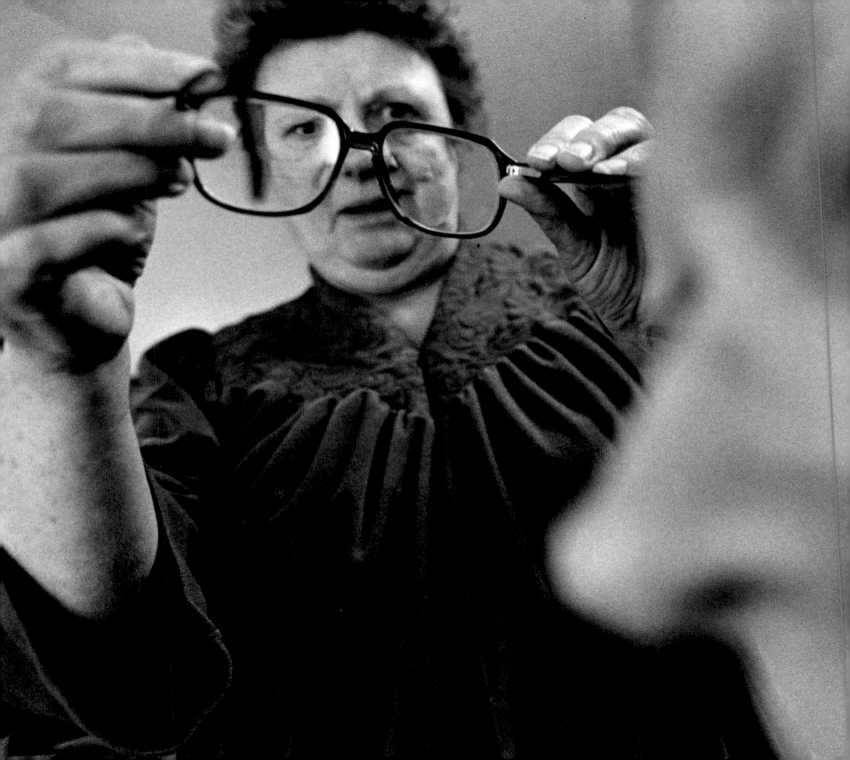

I would just chalk up paranoia as one of those things which is basic to Alzheimer's people. The feeling of frustration, the feeling of having missed something. It's real big, it's heavy. We miss a lot of things and there are times when I feel like people are plotting against me, mainly because I don't hear anything from them, I don't hear good words from them all the time, I'm not doing what I want to do all the time. I think paranoia, if I'm reading things right, almost has to be something that's very basic to living with Alzheimer's.

The caregivers are doing their darndest—they want to be like any other people, and they deserve their moments, their times—their times away from us, because it can be very tedious. We can be very tedious. I can be very tedious, and I'm aware of that.

Sometimes we get to be very demanding—when things don't come the way they should, when they could, I very often get a little bit angry. I do feel very often that I'm being overlooked and I do feel very often that things have passed by me.

It's something you can't ride out of, you can't walk away from, and I guess we owe it to everybody concerned to know that we do love them and sometimes we do feel cheated, mad, or somehow underappreciated.

It's just that when you lose the most valuable things in your life—your career, not to mention making money, and other fool things like that—and just the feeling that you are inferior somehow—that you're no good anymore. I feel that way and I don't want to feel that way—don't want anybody else to feel that way, but I do.

There are times when I feel the whole world is cheating me—out to get me—mainly on things where I don't understand correctly or sensibly. It's sometimes very hard to realize the sacrifice they're making for us. I certainly have no right to criticize anybody, but I just hope that my family and friends do realize that being an Alzheimer's person is—just a little bit of hell. And I do feel cheated—other people do get cheated too out of much of their lives—I can think about paraplegics and other people who are in much worse shape—at least that's one way to look at it—it could be an awful lot worse.

Feeling sorry for ourselves I do imagine is a perfectly normal part of having Alzheimer's because your care-givers are not you and you're not them—they can do their darndest and sometimes we will feel very put upon no matter what.

There are days when you feel so very bad about the whole thing that somehow you wish you could just go away and cry.

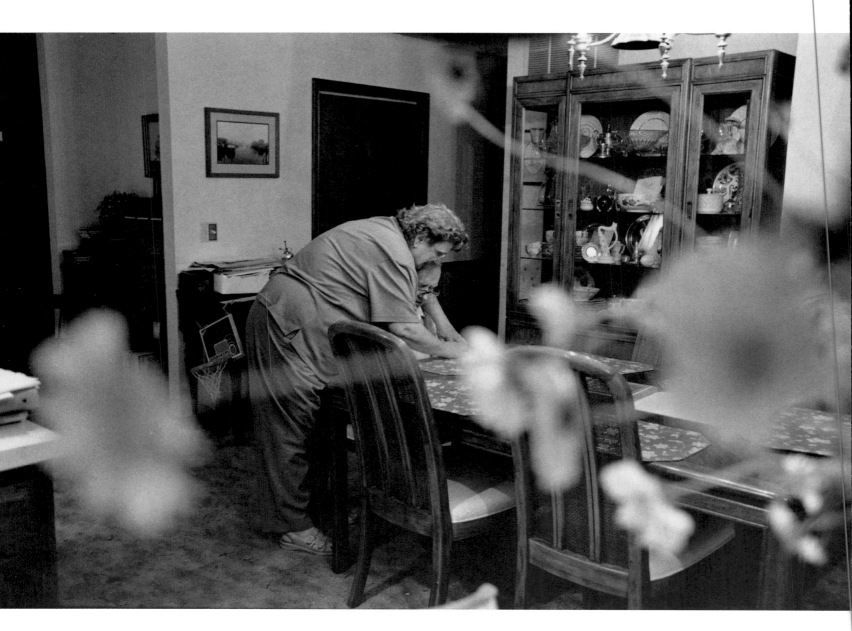

My wife very often wonders why I do things and say things I do and I'll be darned if I know.

Sometimes you remember things that you've said that you wish you had not said. And on the other hand, probably you didn't actually say it. You just thought you said it.

I'm trying to make the point about Alzheimer's people—they make an awful lot of mistakes—just try to bear with them and correct them gently—if you fuss at somebody with Alzheimer's for any length of time—there's no sense in fussing at 'em anyhow—because I don't believe they'll understand what the problems are.

My advice to people who are caregivers is that . . . really . . . just keep things under control. Keep things easy to understand—not baby language or something like that. Don't talk down to us. Don't get mad when we forget things—because getting mad is part of Alzheimer's. We kick ourselves probably all the time. Certainly for myself, I get tired of asking: When are we going to do this? What is going to be this thing? My wife will tell me and a couple of days—well a couple of minutes—later I will have forgotten what day it's going to be. It frustrates everybody. On the other hand, we don't want to keep our mouths shut all the time. We want to help. We want to be part of something, and being a part of something when you don't know what you're being a part of, is—lets call it interesting. Frustrating is not a nice word.

We just make a lot of mistakes in what we say and we don't see a lot of things that we should see, and we think sometimes we see things we haven't really seen—they're not there. There are spooks in all kinds of businesses and endeavors, and there are spooks in Alzheimer's too.

There have been times when I was absolutely sure that one team had won, the way I look at it, and somehow or another, they hadn't won at all, as my wife tells me as she looks at the paper and she can tell these things and sometimes I can't . . .

There have been times when I've thought that I got the signals right and that the Dodgers won or else the Raiders won but somehow it fools you. I'd be absolutely sure something had happened and it really hadn't happened. It kinda gets old after a while, but the wonderful things that I think happened probably have not happened, and probably never will happen—I really don't know. This is very deflating when you think you have discovered something, and you think it's kind of inter-esting or unusual, and then you'll hear, not long after that, that it just never happened.

When you have Alzheimer's there are a lot of things you have to get used to. One of these things is just being dead wrong. I've learned not to argue with anybody about the outcome, say, of a baseball game. I have a hard time knowing, sometimes, whether it's real or not. Even things that you have seen very recently and very clearly, you may not have seen at all. You just think you saw them. You dreamed you saw them.

I remember the University of—somewhere—hospital, I got so agitated that they had to strap me down. Oh God, did I hate that. I got so excited and so mad that I think I may have even hurt myself. I was kicking and screaming. I was doing everything wrong. It's hard when it's you going through all this, especially if people don't communicate with you. They didn't do a very good job of explaining what they were supposed to be doing, and doing it gently. In other words, they were too clinical about it. And I remember that night as one of the very worst nights in all the time I've lived.

My wife has gone to a coffee klatch with her girl friends—which is perfectly all right—but one of the first things that I noticed as Alzheimer's began to creep up was that—when my wife was playing bridge—this was a couple of years ago—and I was at home and I got really really upset and biggest reason was I couldn't contact anybody. I really don't know how to operate little things like—even the TV, radio—everything seemed to be wrong that day. And it's a day I'll never forget. I was so lonely and so frustrated that I called the police to show me where my house was or show me if somebody was home.

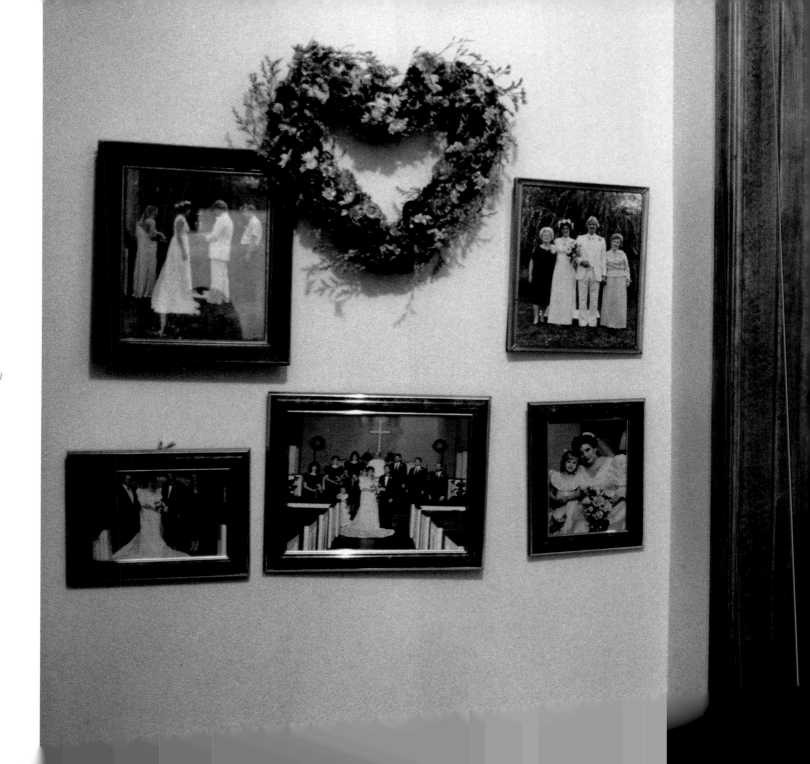

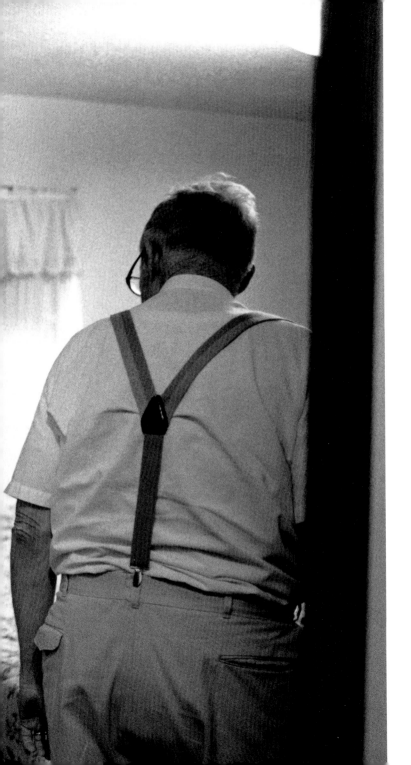

One thing I do have to say though is I'm very glad we
have pictures. My wife remembers specific things but
I really can't do that—I have to be reminded.

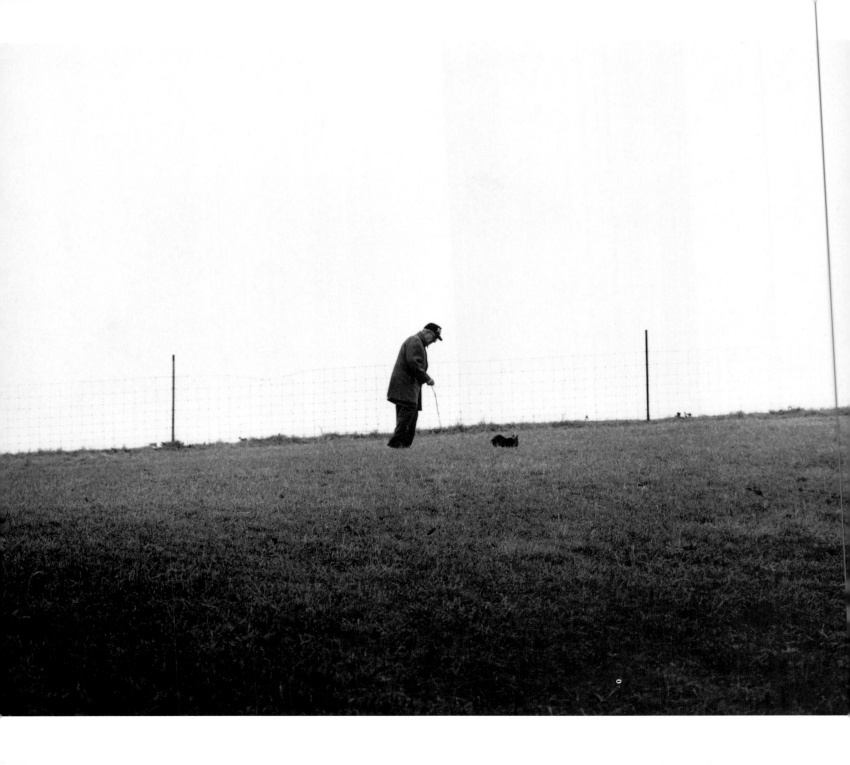

As I ramble around, there are some things that probably
ought to be said that I'm sure I haven't said. But, my
philosophizing for this day is about finished. I can't
imagine there's enough tape in there for any more.
And what's more, I think I've said all that I can say.

The one thing I know though is the dog is with me and
when the dog is with me I at least have some solace,
even if I don't know the way.

I HAVE WORKED in Alzheimer's disease research for eleven years at the Neurological Disorders Clinic (previously the Memory Disorders Clinic) at Duke University Medical Center in Durham, North Carolina. My primary job is the coordination of clinical drug trials for the Joseph and Kathleen Bryan Alzheimer's Disease Research Center. My work involves considerable time spent talking with patients and their caregivers. When I first started in this position, my only knowledge of Alzheimer's was the fact that it was a disease that affected memory. My limited knowledge never prepared me for what I was soon to learn: the reality of Alzheimer's disease goes far beyond both the definition of the clinical diagnosis of Alzheimer's and the general perception which the American public has of this illness.

My teachers were the caregivers who lived *The 36-Hour Day*.[†] The caregivers were spouses, children, siblings, nieces, nephews, and friends. I listened, absorbed, and tried to imagine myself in their place. I thought I was well educated about the disease until I met Cary Henderson in 1989 when he came to the clinic to participate in a drug trial.

Cary, his wife, Ruth, and I met regularly (every other week) for five months from April to September

Afterword

[†] *The 36-Hour Day: A Guide to Caring for Persons with Alzheimer's Disease, Related Dementing Illnesses and Memory Loss in Later Life*, by Nancy L. Mace and Peter V. Rabins.

of 1989 and, thereafter, every three months until February of 1993. We often talked about his frustrations, his depressions, and his paranoias. In January of 1992 Cary told me, "People don't want to talk with me." Cary wanted to talk to people and to listen to them, not only because he thought he could teach them (being a retired history professor), but also because he wanted to learn from them. Through Cary I realized how much I did not know about the reality of living with Alzheimer's disease day after day after day. Over the years the caregivers' perspectives were invaluable in educating me in the reality of living with one diagnosed with Alzheimer's disease, but it was Cary who taught me what it truly meant to live with this affliction; and it was Cary's "Musings," published in the *Duke Caregiver*, that was the impetus for one of the first patient and caregiver support groups in the country.

Even though Cary wrote, "I really would like to know what other people with Alzheimer's feel and what their experiences are," he was hesitant at first to agree to meet with other patients when I first approached him and Ruth about the idea. I can understand his reluctance. Were Cary's experiences with Alzheimer's universal? Were there really others who lived in such a strange world within their own minds, or was Cary the only one? Would he appear more foolish or "stupid" than he already felt? No matter what the consequences might have been, Cary agreed to meet with other patients, and the first casual meeting of the minds was on July 14, 1992. The patients who participated came with the knowledge that they had one common bond—a memory problem which their doctors had diagnosed as Alzheimer's disease. What they left with that day was a feeling of camaraderie. According to Cary, he did not feel alone anymore. In retrospect, what happened that day can be summarized in one word—support. After introducing Cary and Ruth to the other patients and caregivers and explaining again Cary's intent for the meeting, Cary asked his first question. "I start talking to my wife and right in the middle of talking to her I forget what I was going to tell her. Do any of you ever do this?" Agreement echoed throughout the room. He asked his second question. "I go to the kitchen to get some coffee and return to the den without it because I could not remember what I had gone to the kitchen for. Do you do this?" Heads nodded and faces relaxed. Within minutes, Cary repeated his first question, and the others responded as if they had heard it for the first time. For two hours the patients talked with each other and asked "do you do

96

this" questions back and forth (and over and over). Not only was there a sense of relief and release for the patients; there was also a new sense of awareness for the caregivers.

There are people (and organizations) who express doubt about the usefulness of support groups for Alzheimer's patients. I am sorry that this is so; yet I can understand their doubt. So often in diagnosing and treating any illness, it is the patient who becomes lost or forgotten in the process. This is true more often than not with an Alzheimer's patient. We ask them a question but rely on the caregiver to respond. We want their history but listen to the secondary source. As anyone who works with an Alzheimer's patient knows, this is necessary to do, but, in doing so, should we allow necessity to isolate the patient from us? Families want a diagnosis, but, if the diagnosis is Alzheimer's disease, many caregivers prefer to not tell the patients; or some caregivers will allow a memory problem to be acknowledged but will ask that the word "Alzheimer's" not be used. Alzheimer's is a difficult diagnosis to hear, but no matter how difficult it may be, we need to think of the patient first. This is what Cary needed and

wanted, and this is what Cary achieved. He achieved this not only for himself but also for other Alzheimer's patients.

For over six years patients and caregivers have been meeting monthly at the Neurological Disorders Clinic because of Cary Henderson. For the first thirty minutes the patients and caregivers meet jointly to share news, to celebrate birthdays and anniversaries, to brag about new grandchildren, and to make plans for future meetings. Afterwards the patients and caregivers meet separately with facilitators. Even though some of the patients need to be reminded every time about the purpose of the group, they share a bond that remains constant. Together they find strength and courage in being able to say "I have Alzheimer's disease." They acknowledge and grieve their losses. They laugh at themselves but ask that others not laugh or make fun of them. They unselfishly give of their time and energy to educate others about their disease. They find comfort in being able to be themselves. For others living with Alzheimer's disease who do not have such a place to go, I hope Cary's words can offer them the same solace and camaraderie he has given to this group.

SARAH VANN WYNE
Duke University Medical Center
Durham, North Carolina
August 1998

97

Acknowledgments

CARY SMITH HENDERSON:

My wife has been an absolutely wonderful help and she's given up a lot for me and I'm very very grateful for that and my daughter is editing my memoirs, taking charge of my recording and things like that. [Note: Cary's acknowledgments were transcribed from his tapes recorded in 1991–92.]

NANCY ANDREWS:

My sincere thanks to the entire photography staff at *The Washington Post* for their continued support. Special thanks to my Picture Editor Michel duCille, Assistant Managing Editor Joseph Elbert, former Managing Editor Robert Kaiser, and Executive Editor Leonard Downie for providing the creative atmosphere at the paper which allows for projects such as this one. Many thanks to colleagues who provided comment on the text and photographs: Carol Guzy, Mary-Ellen Phelps Deily, Kathryn Jourdan, Leslie Aun, Michael McClain and Marileen Maher.

Most importantly I thank all the members of the Henderson family who opened their lives to me and my camera. I give special thanks to Jackie Main for inviting me to join her and her father in this special project, and for her artful eye throughout the editing process. I thank Ruth Henderson for her eloquent work and her patience at having a camera pointed in her direction. I owe my greatest debt to Cary Henderson, whose revealing words guided my photography which allowed me to take a unique picture of Alzheimer's. Cary was not an unknowing subject. Through his journal, I know that Cary was at times painfully ashamed of his condition, yet he chose to let me photograph him in order to share his life with others. For this I am grateful.

Ruth Henderson, Jackie Main and I give our warmest thanks to our agent Howard Yoon for his dedication and skill. We thank contributors Lonnie D. Kliever and Sarah Vann Wyne for their fine words. Thanks to Lisa P. Gwyther for being the first to recognize the power of Cary's words and to publish them in the *Duke Caregiver*. Thanks to Dr. Nancy Earl, and support group members at the Neurological Disorders Clinic at Duke University Medical Center for allowing us to make photographs at their meetings.

We thank Eric Newton, Cara Sutherland, and the staff at the Newseum in Arlington, Virginia, for exhibiting this work.

Special thanks to the staff at Southern Methodist University Press who shared our vision for this book: Keith Gregory, director; Kathryn Lang, senior editor; and Freddie Jane Goff, production managing editor; and to Tom Dawson of Tom Dawson Graphic Design.

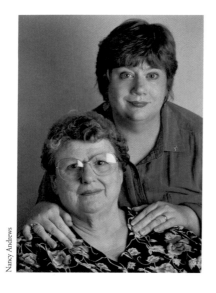

Nancy Andrews

JACKIE HENDERSON MAIN was born in New Jersey and grew up in Harrisonburg, Virginia. She earned a master's degree in counseling psychology from James Madison University. Her professional experience has included work with substance abusers, the mentally ill, and the frail elderly. She is currently a counselor with the Virginia State Department of Rehabilitative Services. She and her husband, David, live in Charlottesville, Virginia, with their two sons, Elijah and Andrei.

RUTH HENDERSON was born in Union City, New Jersey. She is a graduate of Queens College in Charlotte, North Carolina. In 1989 she retired from teaching eighth grade English to be able to care full time for her husband. In addition to caregiving, she is an active volunteer with the Alzheimer's Association's Shenandoah Valley Chapter in Harrisonburg, Virginia.

NANCY ANDREWS, thirty-four, has made pictures for *The Washington Post* for eight years. In 1998 she was named Newspaper Photographer of the Year by the University of Missouri and the National Press Photographer's Association in the 55th Annual Pictures of the Year competition. She has received more than seventy-five professional awards for her work and is a frequent lecturer. In 1994 HarperCollins published her first book, *FAMILY: A Portrait of Gay and Lesbian America*.

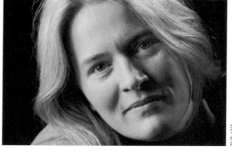

Bill O'Leary

Nancy has participated in group exhibitions and had several solo shows, the largest being at The Corcoran Gallery of Art in Washington, D.C. In 1993 she was awarded a visual arts fellowship from the Virginia Museum of Fine Arts. Prior to coming to the *Post*, Nancy worked at *The Free Lance-Star* in Fredericksburg, Virginia. She is a 1986 graduate of the University of Virginia with a degree in economics.

She currently lives in Arlington, Virginia, with her partner, Sandra Gillis.